CUT THE CRAP

The No-Nonsense Plan for a Healthy Body and Mind

RUTH FIELD

sphere

SPHERE

First published in Great Britain in 2015 by Sphere

1 3 5 7 9 10 8 6 4 2

A CIP catalogue record for this book
is available from the British Library.

ISBN 978-0-7515-5674-2

Typeset in Bembo by M Rules
Printed and bound in Great Britain by
Clays Ltd, St Ives plc

Papers used by Sphere are from well-managed forests
and other responsible sources.

MIX
Paper from
responsible sources
FSC
www.fsc.org FSC® C104740

Sphere
An imprint of
Little, Brown Book Group
100 Victoria Embankment
London EC4Y 0DY

An Hachette UK Company
www.hachette.co.uk

www.littlebrown.co.uk

Dad, this one's got your name on it

CONTENTS

PART 3 SAPS DECONSTRUCTED

PART 4 CONSOLIDATION AND CELEBRATION

WHO IS THE GRIT DOCTOR?

I am The Grit Doctor. I am a ruthless, no-nonsense motivator who will force you to get to grips with your poor eating habits and cut the crap from your diet – and mind – for good. I am the voice you will tune into when you are feeling weak and ineffectual and the one who will help you ignore the deafening call of the Dairy Milk. I will whisper in your ear, YOU FAT BITCH when you are contemplating one more roast potato.

Once you learn to understand and enjoy the voice of The Grit Doctor, it won't be long before you can tune into it whenever you choose to and use it to push yourself forward when you might otherwise give up. The voice of The Grit Doctor is what you've been missing in your life. You just didn't know it until now.

THE CRAP-CUTTING PLEDGE

I, _____ , do solemnly declare that from this day forth I shall give up all diets of any description. I will practise instead mindful, healthy eating until such practice becomes as ingrained a habit as brushing my teeth so that I can devote my energies to other more important shit. I will vow to move more – every day – and to see this as a vital discipline to acquire. I will learn how to do all this through listening to and obeying The Grit Doctor at all times while maintaining my sense of humour.

INTRODUCTION

Food dominates our lives. There is no subject more important, more urgent, more pressing on our minds and our bellies than food. And, yet, when it comes to this essential topic, we are *full of crap*: from the crap we mindlessly shove down our cakeholes while glued to the telly, to the crappy diets we yo-yo between *ad infinitum*, to the crap the media feed us (and we swallow) which fosters our collective paranoia about our bodies and the food we put into them. This is an area over which – in theory at least – we have so much control, but more often than not are left feeling utterly powerless, spent, confused ... and hungry. The Grit Doctor has had enough. Enough of being told that it is bad to eat carbs and good to eat egg-white omelettes. Enough of being force-fed endless images of celebrities stick-thin just six weeks after giving birth. Enough of banal reality TV shows and mean-spirited magazines pointing the finger at people's bodies and inviting us to laugh at and judge them. IT IS ALL CRAP. It is distracting us from the real issues, the important stuff about food that actually matters: from food labelling to portion size, from sugar addiction to our insatiable appetite for processed foods – issues that demand our scrutiny so that we can make better food choices for ourselves and our increasingly porky children. Deep? Gritty? You betcha, bitches.

OLLY'S FOOD DIARY

Those of you who read *Run Fat B!tch Run* will remember that my husband Olly was a guinea pig for my brutal training regime. Well, poor Olly is back in the hot seat. I have always baulked at his diet, but in fairness it is probably the typical lifestyle of a sedentary, overweight male in his late thirties: too much junk and not enough exercise. I've always told myself there is nothing I can do because I have enough on my plate dealing with our twins' and my own healthy eating, without worrying about what Olly is eating all day. And, I always cook for me and Olly in the evening, so I know he's getting at least one (but possibly only one) good meal each day. He often skips breakfast and I know he eats rubbish all day at work – the empty McDonald's containers, Haribo packets and Twix wrappers littering the car are proof. Once, when we were staying at my parents' house and he was on his way back there from court for supper, I saw him on the CCTV intercom on the doorstep shoving a Big Mac down his gob! A 'modest starter' he later claimed in his defence.

Anyway, Olly was at his twenty-year school reunion and found he couldn't get out of the group photo (or Photoshop it afterwards). The result was heinous, or so he tells me. He was genuinely shocked and upset at how fat he was next to his contemporaries; he has refused to show me this photograph but he was really disgusted by it and he realised, in looking at it, how out of shape he had become and particularly how much *more* out of shape he was than his old classmates. I questioned why this hadn't happened with any other photos and then I realised he hates having his photo taken and always avoids it by, of course, being the one on the other side of the lens. And he deletes immediately any shots I do take of him. The camera doesn't lie. (Actually it does, to the tune of an extra 9 lb I think.) Whatever, it is desperately unforgiving and can in an instant shatter any illusions you may have about your frame: if you are fat, you will look fat in a photo.

This awful photograph has become his catalyst, his 'reason', the grain of motivation upon which The Grit Doctor has pounced. His vanity got the better of him and I am just the person to capitalise on his fear and turn it into something positive, to help rid him of some terrible eating habits. Forever. And how convenient that right now I am writing a book preaching the benefits of cutting out crap from your diet. He will be my proof and – hopefully – your inspiration. Actually, there's a personal bonus too – how hot is he going to look with a six pack? Finally, the arm-candy husband I always dreamed of . . .

EXERCISE

Photographic grit-fest

Dig out your favourite photograph of yourself. Chances are, it will be one where you were either at your thinnest or taken at such a flattering angle that you at least *look* thin. For those married women out there, seek out a wedding photograph – I'll hazard a guess almost all of you lost weight for the big day. How successful was the diet that helped you achieve that skinny frame? Look at the photo and then at yourself in the mirror for the answer. You thought that 'miracle diet' was the Holy Grail but look at how badly it has let you down. Now dig out a photo of yourself that you are ashamed of. That you hate. If you have a habit of deleting all 'fat photos' then the time has come to get a special one taken. Let your other half in on the secret – or your best mate or flatmate. No special mirror poses (stomach tucked in etc.), numerous retakes or Instagram filters: this is supposed to make you squirm, so the grittier the better. Grittify everything. Take a series from all angles and then keep the most horrible one.

Look, this exercise is designed to motivate you into action, not depress you into suicide, so stop feeling sorry for yourself and look on the bright side. This photo is going to be your catalyst. If it worked for my stubborn husband, it can work for you too. This fat bitch is going to morph back into the best version of herself, while abandoning the dieting merry-go-round and getting a healthy heart and fit, toned frame to boot. With bags of energy and resourcefulness she never knew she had. What's not to love?

Stick the photo on your mirror or fridge as a gritty reminder of what you genuinely look like pre-slap and Spanx, or, for grit fiends, make it your screensaver (all screens please) to bring you straight back to reality whenever you are tempted to reach for a crisp packet, deluded that you are actually looking pretty hot today (fully made up, a few glasses of wine down, pouting at yourself in a 'thin' bar loo mirror). No weeping please, this is vital fuel for your grit tank. If it serves to divert you away from the cake tin or vino bottle and outside for a brisk walk it has served you well.

PART 1

THE INHERENT
MADNESS OF DIETS

1

DIETING DELUSIONS EXPOSED

We are living in a crazy dieting age. Diets and dieters are *everywhere*. When we are not hooked on the latest dieting fad ourselves, you can guarantee that someone in our family, among our closest friends, on the bus, at the swings, in the park toilets for faaaark's sake, is. And I want to scream about it from the top of my lungs: 'WHAT IS WRONG WITH US ALL?! ARE WE COMPLETELY MAD?'

There is a group of lovely women who have coffee in the café where I write, every week after they drop their kids off at school; they are sitting beside me right now. Dieting is always high on their chat agenda. One of them is on the 5:2, another on some wildly restrictive carbohydrate percentage ratio diet – and they discuss the highs and lows of their eating regimes at great length while munching on pastries and sipping lattes. Educated, interesting women spending their precious time and energy discussing diets while eating crap. Needless to say, in the year or so that I have been coming to this café, none of these women have remotely changed shape.

You may be asking yourself who does this Grit Doctor woman think she is? Well, unlike your average diet book, I don't pretend to have created the magical elixir juice recipe that is going to be the answer to all your prayers. I am not promising miracles, quick fixes or fancy solutions. I am just an ordinary woman, angry at ever being made to feel that stick-thin is something worth aspiring to; a woman who wasted her late teens and early twenties half starved to death and very unhappy, existing on a diet of rice cakes and gin. A woman who, since those dark days, has successfully maintained roughly the same weight – save for pregnancy – while never going on a diet. How? By eating normally and exercising regularly so that I can get on with the rest of my life.

THE GRIT DOCTOR WILL SEE YOU NOW

Q: If you are not offering anything special, why do I need this book?

A: Oh, you need it. If you are still getting seduced by diets, if you are overweight and feel trapped and overwhelmed by food, or if you are at a normal weight but just terribly unhealthy, eating way too much crap and with no control over your family's eating habits, then you have come to the right place. The Grit Doctor is here to whip you and your kitchen into shape.

Here's the thing: commitment and common sense – The Grit Doctor's twin tenets – are all that is required for you to create a healthy lifestyle and maintain a normal weight *for the rest of your life*. And just imagine what you could do if you were free from the chains of the dieting merry-go-round. If weight issues and food debacles no longer dominated your life. If you were more or less within the right weight range, *for you*, and no longer had to waste precious time and energy worrying about it. Think how happy, free and energised you would be.

Every diet book starts with the basic premise that most diets don't work, but *this one* is different, and then proceeds to be restrictive and prescriptive in the same way as all the others, just presented differently. The only eating pattern that genuinely is not a diet is one that has no restrictions on what you can eat and when. The challenge lies in educating ourselves into forging new habits to such a profound extent that we are more likely to make better choices *most of the time*[1]. I eat all sorts of food. I love red meat, barbecues, curries, bacon sarnies, pizza, red wine, gin, fish and chips, roast dinners, lasagne – to name but a few less healthy

---

1 In Grit Doctor speak, 'most of the time' = 80% of the time.

options. But I also love fish, green vegetables, quinoa, fruit, brown rice, wholemeal bread and – most importantly – I love being fit and healthy. So I choose to try and eat a balanced diet *most of the time*, and when I do eat junk I make up for it over the next few days by eating more healthily and exercising more energetically. No restrictions, no bans, no limits on any of it – particularly the exercise.

THE GRIT DOCTOR SAYS

The notion that we already have everything we need to lose weight and be healthy renders an entire industry redundant, which is why no diet will ever reveal this simple truth.

One thing that is strikingly obvious is that the dieting industry is *massive*. In the UK, it's estimated to be worth more than £2 billion per year[2]; in America, it makes over $60 billion per year[3]. For such a 'successful' industry (i.e. one raking in vast sums of cash), it is also true to say that it is a huge *fail* from the consumer's perspective. For two reasons: 1) because while the dieting industry

2 '5:2 is just the latest: Britain's diet industry is worth £2 billion, so why do we buy into it?' Susan Elkin, *Independent*, 1 August 2013
3 http://www.marketresearch.com/Marketdata-Enterprises-Inc-v416/Weight-Loss-Status-Forecast-8016030/

grows, it is doing so under the shadow of an obesity pandemic, and 2) because around 97 per cent of dieters fail. For every three dieters who succeed in losing weight, this means that there are *ninety-seven* others who don't – and who probably feel like total losers as a result. How can an industry making $60 billion each year have a 97 per cent outright failure rate? How is it that as a society we find these statistics acceptable? Why are there not government health warnings on the spines of diet books alerting hopefuls to this pitiful evidence? Why are we not holding the dieting industry to account?[4] Would we buy a dress if it only had a three per cent chance of making it past its first party without falling apart at the seams? Would we opt for a caesarean-section if the operation had a 97 per cent failure rate? Err, no. So why is it that we keep coming back for more?

The answer is in the maths. It is the high failure rate that ensures the enduring success of the industry because customers keep coming back for another shot when the last diet didn't work out. And why do we not give up in the face of almost certain – and repeated – failure? Because the overarching narrative of the dieting industry is that we are inadequate, and only it has the cure for our failings. And that once cured (i.e. thin) we will have a handsome husband, beautiful children, money, success and power to boot. So, the chance to slim down – no matter how slim that

4 Susie Orbach, psychologist and author of *Fat is a Feminist Issue*, has been threatening to sue Weight Watchers International, which she views as symbolic of the whole dieting industry. She claims the 97% recidivism rate contravenes the Trade Descriptions Act 1968.

chance really is – becomes more than just a number on a set of scales in the world of weight-loss marketing: it becomes the answer to all of life's problems.[5] The Holy Grail itself.

Our frenetic yo-yoing between deranged diets helps cultivate a language of panic about both weight loss and food: Why have I lost only 2 lb this week despite existing on kale juice and fresh air? If I eat that cake I will never fit into that LBD on Saturday. Why can't I control myself? I NEED CHOCOLATE. Rooted in the short term, and tied to a spurious number on the scales, the dialogue around food becomes emotionally charged and confusing at best, dishonest and dangerous at worst.

The diet industry is bending over backwards to blind us to the basic facts that eating less crap and exercising more is all you need to know to maintain a healthy weight. Why? Because no one makes any money out of empowering individuals to take responsibility for themselves. The diet industry thrives on having us feel powerless, out of control and unable to succeed without them and their magic pill, potion or secret combination of food groups that will literally melt away our fat . . . and fears.

THE GRIT DOCTOR SAYS

If the dieting industry worked, there would be no return customers and no profit – so failure is its

---

5 *Separating Fact From Fiction In The Age Of Obesity* by Courtney E. Martin

raison d'être, its central truth. And that is deeply screwed up.

After decades of complex, contradictory and profit-driven messaging on the part of the multi-billion-pound dieting industry, it has become almost impossible to believe that the power to be healthy is so simple and already exists within us all. And so we choose over and over again not to believe it, not to trust our basic instincts, not to trust our sound judgement, but instead to believe that carbs after 6 p.m. must be fatal to our waistline; that it is, in fact, sane and healthy to lose 7 lb in seven days on a juice-only diet; that cutting out major food groups is a necessary evil to be endured in our desperate quest for an unattainable level of 'thin' – the default remedies for all our ills, upsets and disappointments. Dieting exists entirely in the language of false promises and delusional expectations, and it feeds on our deepest insecurities and fears.

A SUCCESSFUL DIET

What is the measure of success in a diet anyway? How do we define it? Are those three per cent of dieters 'successful' because they lost 7 lb in seven days on a juice-only diet? What if you were 7 lb lighter for a party, but two weeks later you are 4 lb heavier than before you got juiced? Does that make your juice diet a failure? What if you are one of those people who have lost loads of weight on various diets during different periods of your life, but are now many pounds heavier than you were before you jumped on the dieting bandwagon? What if you are now on the 5:2 diet – the current fad as I write, which will almost certainly be 'so over' by the time you are reading this in print – and are finding it to be working? Have you considered that you are basically resigning yourself to living on a starvation diet for 104 days out of every year? Would it not be preferable instead to eat normally every day – just less crap and more green veg, a bit less fat and sugar with some exercise in between?

Diets can only ever succeed in the short term. You win when the scales tip in your favour, yet lose as soon as you stop the diet and go back to eating 'normally' again. But no more. Because The Grit Doctor has had enough. She is a powerful voice who will help you locate your own inner grit: an essential tool in your quest for a healthier lifestyle. Bad news for the dieting gravy train and great news for your waistline.

THE GRIT DOCTOR TRANSLATES SOME POPULAR DIETS

Alkaline Ash – Steal vast quantities of litmus paper from your kids' school chemistry lab for peeing on to make sure your body's pH is bang on the money.

Paleo – Because evolution never really happened did it?

Sugar Free – Eat only, err, meat and fats, sugarkins. Beyond deranged.

5:2 – Live like an anorexic for two days a week and lose weight. Surprise, surprise.

Dukan – Don't. Can't.

Atkins – Eat protein and fat and enjoy smelly breath, insomnia and constipation. WARNING: Heart attacks and kidney failure possible. Bad health guaranteed.

The Zone – Remove any joy and spontaneity from mealtimes. Get degrees in nutrition and maths so you can get those carb/protein ratios bang on every time. And you'll need to buy back the scales that I'm going to make you give away later, as you'll need them to weigh your food.

South Beach – Atkins renamed, revised and revamped.

Raw Food – How to lose friends and alienate people. Never EVER enjoy a normal meal again.

Juice – Regress to babyhood and allow no solids to pass your lips for a week. WARNING: Expect to faint. A lot. Or die.

Detox – Binge like a fiend and punish yourself afterwards through starvation.

Breatharian – Live on, err, fresh air and sunlight? Guaranteed death if followed successfully.

Fruitarian – Exist only on fruit, vegetables, nuts and seeds. Mmm. Not God's Way.

THE GRIT DOCTOR SAYS

It doesn't take a nutritionist or a scientist to tell you that any eating regime which prescribes excluding entire food groups can be neither sane nor healthy, let alone sustainable or realistic.

EXORCISE YOUR DIET

Anyone currently on a diet, or who has just given up on one, and especially any of you who are always on and off diets, please re-read the previous five pages over and over again until the contents really sink in. Doesn't it make you feel angry? Abused, even? At the very least, taken advantage of? We are bombarded and bamboozled with this message from every media angle available: that 'thin' is the door to paradise and only it (the dieting industry) holds the key. Just dig out your favourite magazine and I guarantee that somewhere on the front cover will be a reference to an actress or some other celeb having found nirvana – a hot, rich husband and a blossoming career – all on account of her shrinking to a size six.

Because we fail on every diet we try – as we are bound to, given the statistics – we become trapped, stuck on the dieting merry-go-round forever, never able to lose weight and maintain it, powerless over an artificially targeted number on a set of scales, while feeling hungry, tired and fed up with ourselves for always falling short. And fat to boot! A ludicrous state of affairs when you consider the facts, don't you think?

THE GRIT DOCTOR SAYS
There *is* a permanent escape from all this nonsense and I will help you find it.

EXERCISE

Close your eyes. You are back at school and in detention. Try to think of a lifestyle pursuit, or any other activity, that you would willingly choose to do if you knew you had a 97 per cent chance of failing at it. Step on that plane? Go to university? Get married? Learn French? Bungee jump? Drive a car? Ask her out on a date? Have that operation?

There is, of course, *nothing* you would willingly do if you knew it had a 97 per cent failure rate. Now open your eyes and write out your lines:

97 per cent of ALL diets FAIL. Anything which has a 97 per cent failure rate is a fool's game.

Write this out 100 times.

When finished, stick it on your fridge or mirror alongside

your fat photo and kiss those ludicrous stats goodbye. FOR-EVER.

WITHIN YOU

Some good news: nestled wi*thin* is the 'you' that you were always supposed to be, shape and weight-wise. This applies even if you are very overweight and the real you is currently hidden beneath a thick layer of subcutaneous fat. This book is designed to help you relocate *that* version of you: the version hidden within, not the Victoria Beckham-esque version or the size six version but the real, healthy you. Because there is an optimum shape and size destined for you alone, waiting to be rediscovered. It is without doubt the healthiest 'you', the version your body functions best at, because it is the one coded into your DNA, as definitive as your height and eye colour.[6] But the important thing you have to accept is that reaching this optimum weight is highly unlikely to result in your suddenly becoming Kate Moss's body double. And denying this truth is part of the reason – perhaps – that you never seem to be able to reach the number you set yourself on the scales, or stay at it for very long.

---

6 Dr Susan Albers, author of *Eating Mindfully: How to End Mindless Eating and Enjoy a Balanced Relationship with Food*, explains: 'According to the "set point" theory . . . your body has a genetically predetermined weight range. Your body tries to keep your weight within that range and will automatically adjust your metabolism and food storage capacity to keep you from losing or gaining weight outside of that range or set point.'

THE GRIT DOCTOR WARNS

Before you breathe an enormous sigh of relief and put your feet up again, confident that it is your DNA or a 'fat gene' at fault for your thick waistline, you are missing the point entirely. Read on.

SIDE EFFECTS OF EXCESSIVE AND YO-YO DIETING

- Exhaustion
- Wreaks havoc with your metabolism
- Makes you fatter long term
- Sinus problems
- Bloodshot eyes
- Gallbladder disease
- Rashes
- Muscle atrophy
- Seizures
- Dehydration
- Fainting
- Acidosis (increased acidity in the blood)
- Constipation
- Irritability

- Depression
- Lower sex drive
- Lack of concentration
- Loss of memory
- Obsessive thoughts
- Bingeing
- Panic attacks
- Heart attacks
- Liver failure
- Kidney failure
- Anorexia, bulimia
- Oh and lest we forget, a 97 per cent chance of FAILURE

THE GRIT DOCTOR SAYS

Dieting is a form of self-harm.

Because we are force-fed images of scantily clad supermodels or gazelle-like celebs on a daily basis and from every imaginable angle – buses, billboards, television-times-a-gazillion-channels, newspapers, Twitter, Facebook – we have come to see super-thin as a normal shape that we can surely attain if only we diet hard enough. Along the way we have forgotten that supermodels are, in fact, genetic freaks; in a global population of however many billion people, you can actually count them. There are more Nobel Peace Prize winners than there are supermodels, for God's sake. This is totally deranging because the reality is we are more likely to come across a UFO than meet someone as freakishly tall and thin as a supermodel in real life. And that's *before* the digital enhancement that further improves, elongates and plumps up their already 'perfect' bodies, creating an impossible standard in the most literal sense. This all suits the media down to a tee, of course, because it fuels the advertising industry, the movie industry and of course the darkest of them all, the dieting industry. And so young girls bingeing on these images continue to waste years of their lives half-starved and depressed about not being thin or beautiful enough. What a colossal waste of their time and energy.

THE GRIT DOCTOR SAYS

Trust me, these celebs and supermodels are on the 5:2, but the '2' refers to their eating days. The rest of the week they are living on a version of the Breatharian Diet with a side order of cosmetic surgery.

EXERCISE

Burn or bag exercise

Dig out all your dieting books, DVDs and scales – anything and everything diet-related. Yes, that does include photos of size-zero celebs pinned to your fridge for 'thinspiration'. And yes, that also includes items of clothing that you are keeping to wear 'someday when I am skinny'. Why? Because both that photo and that dress represent an unattainable level of thin that you are wasting your energy aspiring to. You will never reach that weight and be healthy.

Part of giving up dieting is giving up the dream of an unrealistic shape and accepting the fact that there is a natural healthy weight and shape for you, just waiting to be realised. And it is *beautiful*. Not because some bullshit-media-dictated-ever-changing impossible standard says so. But because it is you. It may be a few pounds less (or more) than you are at the moment, or even a few stone, but it is definitely *not* a size zero. Or a size six, for that matter. Or Gisele.

Trashy magazines also qualify for burning and act as great kindling for the more heavy-duty dieting tomes. Either burn or bag everything. Take the bag to the charity shop without delay or regret. Burn everything else. Do combine this with the crisp-burning exercise on page 168 if you are in a particularly fiery kind of mood.

As with any de-cluttering exercise, once completed, you will feel lighter, freer and ready to tackle the next stage of your crap-cutting mission with gusto.

FATTER FACTS

Although a very serious issue that needs to be addressed, half-starved youngsters are, thank God, at the thinner end of the problem. The majority of us sit at the fatter end. 60 per cent of adult males, 50 per cent of adult females and 25 per cent of our children will be obese by 2050. It is estimated that the annual cost to the NHS of all this fat will reach £9.7 billion by 2050, with wider costs to society estimated to reach £49.9 billion.[7] These factors combine to make the prevention of obesity the major public health challenge for everybody: government, food manufacturers, schools, the NHS, you and me. And it is a challenge that none of us can afford to ignore any longer: fat is fast becoming the new black.

THE GRIT DOCTOR WILL SEE YOU NOW

Q: So, if dieting is so bad, why is it also so bad to be fat? What weight should we be?

---

7 These figures are from the Department of Health's 2007 *Foresight Report* and are now widely argued to have *underestimated* the magnitude of the problem.

A: It's not bad to be fat any more than it is good to
be thin. Good and bad have nothing to do with our
shapes and sizes. The only point of relevance here is
our health. There is incontrovertible evidence that
being overweight, especially being grossly overweight,
has extremely adverse effects on our health. Not
maybe, not possibly, but most definitely. See the lists
on pages 105 and 133 for examples. And while it is
unarguably true that being very underweight is also
dangerously unhealthy, it is far, FAR less common. If
something is so obviously injurious to your health –
like smoking, for example – it would be a strange
thing to ignore its cure when that cure is entirely
within your own power to administer. And while this
is a book which deals primarily with issues affecting
those who are overweight, a more critical, honest and
less emotional approach to the way we feed ourselves
will hopefully help those whose struggles are at the
lighter end of scales too.

If being overweight is stopping you from
participating fully in your life – at work, sexually, at
your Sunday morning kickabout – then focus on
these areas and try to use them as grist for your
healthy eating mill. But I want you to try to give up
feeling defensive or emotional about it. This is where

we are all going wrong. We need to divorce our
emotions from our food to succeed. Get over it. You
are fat, yes? Fine, now let's bloody well do
something about it.

As for the question what weight should you be? In
the absence of a better alternative, and unless you are
a professional bodybuilder, get your BMI measured
using an online calculator and use its weight range
as your guide.[8] If you can get your weight within
that range – and keep it there – you will have
removed all those serious health concerns linked to
obesity.

Aspiring to an unrealistic body shape is the same as targeting a
meaningless number on a set of scales, or panic-buying diet pills,
or making a promise to your other half (as you speed dial
Domino's from the sofa) that you will start that diet on Monday –

8 The Body Mass Index is going to be your guide. Use an online calculator to find out
what it is or go to your GP and get it established. Aim to get to and stay within that range.
Where you choose to remain once within that range is a matter for you and your vanity.
There is a recent trend pointing away from the BMI as the ideal guideline for your healthy
weight range. The theory is that there is a group of 'healthy' obese people for whom it is
not an accurate measurement and who require more sophisticated criteria. For example, a
bodybuilder was shocked to be told by her GP that she was obese according to her BMI
measurement. Both bodybuilder and GP need to be shot. I am writing for the majority for
whom the BMI will do quite nicely thank you very much.

they all miss the point entirely. Healthy weight management isn't about a number, or the fantasy of a minuscule dress size to bolster flagging self-esteem, or getting *somewhere someday* when you have finally won the battle of the bulge and can relax once again and tuck into a scone. It isn't about losing 3 lb a week or four stone in six months for your wedding day only to see it all creep back on after the honeymoon.

It is about making a commitment right now to eating more healthily *for the rest of your days.* It is about cultivating a new relationship with food that is about having more energy, a stronger heart and a longer life: a life where you might get to enjoy your retirement safe from the perils of diabetes, cardiovascular disease and cancer. If you can cut the crap out of your diet, this longer, healthier life will be yours. And the first thing that has to go are the scales. And along with them your attitude to eating and weight management as something that you should measure weekly or daily. Or at all. Start eating well for your life and the right weight and body shape will find you.

THE GRIT DOCTOR SAYS

When you are living your commitment to eating less crap and exercising regularly you will no longer have to think about your weight.

2

THE CRAP-CUTTING WAY

With a healthier lifestyle comes a more considered approach to our food choices, a set of behaviours and an attitude that is about nourishing our hunger, being satisfied and celebrating our bodies. A way of being that enables us to feel fulfilled in all sorts of ways, so we can stop using food as a crutch or an emotional plug. Feeding our feelings can never free us from them, but it sure as shit is a failsafe strategy to ensure we remain overweight. As Geneen Roth writes in her book *Breaking Free From Emotional Eating*: 'Being hungry is like being in love: if you don't know, you're probably not.'[9]

---

9 The Germans have a brilliant word for weight gain due to emotional eating: *kummerspeck*. It means 'grief bacon'. We've all been there, right?

The Grit Doctor's GOLDEN RULE
The only way into this healthier lifestyle is
through the door of regular exercise.

Once regular exercise becomes a way of life, as it must, you may find that your desire to overeat lessens. In days of yore, we ran to fight or escape danger. This 'fight or flight'[10] instinct produces a hormonal cascade that switches off the hunger centre in the brain and our cravings subside – our body is focused on only one thing: fighting or escaping danger. When we run nowadays, of course, the only clear and present danger is the bakery at the top of the road – but our brains are still tricked into shutting down the hunger centre and so the desire to nip in and pick up a cream cake disappears.[11] Exercise further stimulates the hormones responsible for regulating mood, reducing anxiety and making us feel happy, which can also lead to a lessening desire to snack. Plus, it actually pulls stored energy (glucose and fat) out of body tissues, which regulates sugar levels so you don't feel hungry. And it slows down the passage of food in our guts, keeping us feeling fuller for longer.

---

10 The fight or flight response is a physiological reaction that occurs in response to a perceived harmful event, attack, or threat to survival. The adrenal medulla produces a hormonal cascade that results in the secretion of catecholamines, especially norepinephrine and epinephrine.
11 *The No Crave Diet* by Dr Penny Kendall-Reed and Dr Stephen Reed

The practice of regular exercise makes it harder for you to take your body for granted because you come up against all its weaknesses *and* experience its strength; it forces you to confront all of its glorious vulnerabilities and therefore be more actively engaged with its ongoing needs. Which, loosely translated, means you don't want to feed it so much crap any more.

THE GRIT DOCTOR SAYS

A sustainable shift in our food choices is dependent upon improving our attitude to our bodies. The key to unlock that attitude shift is regular exercise.

Everything – our choices, our beliefs, our fears, our dieting delusions – begins with language, so we have to start recognising crap when we read it. Any time you read something that promises you will 'lose *x* number of pounds in *y* number of days', or contains the words 'miracle new diet', you must remember that there is *no such thing*. It is all nonsense. Ideally, you should stop reading it. Full Stop. At the very least, make a conscious effort to stop being seduced by it and start recognising it for the crap it really is.

I'm sure many of you saw the recent 'like a girl' video[12] that

12 http://www.huffingtonpost.co.uk/2014/06/27/like-a-girl-always-empower-women_n_5536393.html

did the rounds on the internet – if you didn't, I recommend checking it out. The short film, made by Always, asks a group of children to act out throwing, running and fighting 'like a girl', and then challenges them to think about why they all – girls and boys alike – did each task badly. Language shapes how we think and behave, so ultimately can transform both. Language is extremely powerful. Which is why we have a responsibility to use it to motivate and inspire, not to belittle, demean or panic-drive us into buying a year's worth supply of chia seeds.

Also tricky on the language front is being told that sugar is the devil and must be banished from our lives, only to be told the following week that fat is the arch-enemy to be avoided at all costs. How on earth are we supposed to know what to believe? And the language surrounding these 'bad' foods is so extreme, so hyped-up, so inaccurate and has such negative connotations it sends us into something approaching a moral panic. Similarly, foods labelled 'healthy' can be far from it and 'low fat' alternatives are more often than not far crappier than their full-fat sisters. 'Diet speak' operates in the language of extremes, which only serves to reinforce unnatural eating patterns and crazily misinformed food choices. The whole industry is built on a big FAT lie, remember? Confusion is its central premise.

Whenever you are tempted back into diet-type behaviour, or you start to believe the current hype, go back to those lines taped up on your fridge and remind yourself of the statistics. As a general rule of thumb, ignore everything you read that contains the word 'diet'. And try to get into the habit of reading this rubbish with your bullshit detector switched ON, as it will otherwise only help to feed a poor attitude to food. As for navigating the mine-field that is food labelling,[13] the only foolproof way to avoid the vast majority of this crap is to cook as much as you possibly can from scratch.

A GRIT DOCTOR REMINDER

There is no miracle cure, no magical combination of food groups, no pill or potion or secret that can melt away your fat and fears.

There is nothing to sweeten the fact that some of this is hard work, and that it requires thought, patience and commitment and being entirely responsible for your body and what you choose to put into it. Every. Day. And that another big part of that responsibility is a commitment to MOVING MORE.

Make no mistake, overweight is fast becoming the new norm — a fact made painfully clear to me when a family of fatsos recently accused me of being 'too thin'. At 5 ft 10 and 10 st 3 lb with a

13 Please sort this out, Dave.

BMI of 21, I am bang on the money weight-wise; it is they who have lost sight of what is normal. As a society we are complicit in this deceit: clothes sizes have got bigger over recent decades[14] which further perpetuates the collective delusion. A fat girlfriend of mine recently told me that she was a size 12 and I nearly burst out laughing. I am a size 12 and she is at least *twice* my size. Although we quite rightly worry about the negative impact being surrounded by images of stick-thin celebs has on our body image, it's still surprisingly easy to delude ourselves that it's *other people* who are overweight – not us.

It strikes me as absurd that despite living in this THIN, THIN, THIN at all costs culture, we are actually getting FAT, FAT, FAT. Somewhere in the middle of those two extremes is where we ALL need to be, free from the crappy idea that thin is any more the answer to our problems than comfort eating a tub of ice-cream. When we are operating in the middle rather than at either end of that crazy see-saw, we ought to no longer feel starved, but satisfied. Bellies full, and with bodies and minds fit for purpose.

GRITTY HOME TRUTHS

Every time you are in the newsagents buying sweets or choco-late because you are *starving* and desperate for a sugar hit,

14 'Vanity sizing' – a phenomenon popularised since the 1970s – is the common practice of assigning smaller sizes to articles of manufactured clothing than is really the case, in order to encourage sales.

remember this: someone else, someone slimmer and fitter than you, was feeling the same way yet chose to eat an apple instead. And then went for a run. That is the unpalatable truth that no one is telling you straight. You need to accept that your being overweight is no one's fault but your own: not your mum's, not your kid's, not your other half's, it is not your genes nor your slow metabolism. It falls fairly and squarely on your own shoulders. And the reason you are fat is because you eat too much crap and don't move enough. Sure, maybe your mother and father ate a lot of crap too and set you a bad example. Maybe they set you off on a sugar-loaded road, and your metabolism has become sluggish as a result; maybe lack of exercise has become a way of life that feels impossible to transform. I get that you may feel powerless and perhaps angry at what I am saying.

But the important point is always to look at what we *can* change. If you are fat because of *you*, and no one else, then you have the power to change that. It is a useful exercise to distinguish between those things you can exert some control over from those that you cannot and therefore must accept about yourself. For example:

EXERCISE

I can't change my DNA

I can't change the size and width of my hip bones and shoulders

I can't change the fact that I am shit at tennis

I can't change that I love chocolate.

But . . .

I can choose not to put that chocolate into my mouth every time I crave it

I can choose not to have seconds

I can stop believing what the media and diet industry tells me is the 'right' body shape

I can choose not to let the fact that I have no hand–eye co-ordination stop me from starting a Zumba class

Ultimately, understanding those distinctions and taking action where you can will yield massive results over time, for both your mental and physical health, whatever your circumstances or your genetic predisposition or your big bones. So no more excuses or dwelling on the unalterable facts, all right? Good. Let's crack on.

THE GRIT DOCTOR WARNS

If you genuinely consider yourself to be an exception to all this, and believe there's a medical reason why you're overweight, see a real doctor and if necessary stop reading this book until you have the truth confirmed.

The good news is that once you accept responsibility, you begin to realise that you do have all the power to change things – to reverse the damage and undo that decade of cream-cake-as-a-daily-staple type eating. And know too that it may take another decade to undo. You have the rest of your life to work on this, so don't panic yourself into over-the-top-diet-style mode and decide to eat only rice cakes for the rest of the day to get a head start. This way madness and failure lies. And The Grit Doctor wants you to win. So read on, make a cuppa if you will and have a small slice of cake if that's your thing at this time of day – go on, it's not a trick, just cut a piece that is half the size of your normal portion. And eat it slowly. And resolve to do the same next time.[15] Start becoming more mindful[16] about what is passing through your cakehole. Bingo. On the road to recovery already.

THE GRIT DOCTOR SAYS

There is no lifestyle worthy of aspiration that would have us not eat cake, and I'm talking about *real* cake here, not the worthy gluten/sugar/joy-free shit that masquerades as cake.

---

15 DON'T GO BACK FOR SECONDS.

16 Whether it is called intuitive eating, mindful eating, or thoughtful eating, it is essentially the process of basing eating behaviour on physiological cues as opposed to environmental or emotional factors. That is, listening to what your body is telling you rather than stuffing sweets in your gob to cure the loneliness you feel.

'MINDFULNESS', TRANSLATED BY THE GRIT DOCTOR

Simply put, when it comes to food, and especially if you are the sort of person who can put away a whole packet of biscuits and not know how it happened, always think before you put something into your mouth. Train yourself into this habit.

EXERCISE

Some useful questions to ask

'Am I really hungry? No, really?'

'Why am I crying my way into the newsagents to buy enough chocolate to sink a ship?'

'What am I doing?'

'Am I feeling sad? Bored? Tired? Frustrated? How is eating going to solve this?'

'Am I in an Enid Blyton novel? No. Then why am I standing in front of an open fridge door in my nightie, looking for a midnight snack?'

'Is what I am about to put into my mouth going to nourish my body?'

'Am I about to devour sugar-riddled junk food designed to give me a delirious high followed by a crashing low, making me crave more of the stuff like a deranged drug addict?'

In short: STEP AWAY FROM THE DOUGHNUTS.

THE GRIT DOCTOR SAYS

It matters less *what* questions you ask than that you just start asking yourself stuff to establish whether or not you are *genuinely* hungry. It is a habit that, once bedded-in, makes it almost impossible for crap to slip down your gob unnoticed any longer.

Cutting the crap does not mean that you can never again enjoy eating unhealthy foods. It is always possible to make a positive choice to eat something unhealthy when unhealthy eating is no longer the norm, i.e. eating unhealthily is no longer a mindless bad habit that you don't acknowledge or take responsibility for. If you are fat, guaranteed there is too much mindless cake-gobbling going on in your life and not enough considered eating. So, the aim of the game is to think your way into making better, healthier choices *most of the time*.[17]

17 Reminder: in Grit Doctor speak, 'most of the time' = 80% of the time.

THE GRIT DOCTOR SUMMARISES

Less compulsion, more informed choice is the name of the game.

THE GRIT DOCTOR WILL SEE YOU NOW

Q: Easier said than done!

A: You are right. One of the things we must relearn is to recognise hunger cues and eat to feed only those – not gorge endlessly as a reaction to all of our other appetites. Food can only ever satisfy our hunger, it cannot meet any of our other needs. We need to learn how to distinguish between these and one of the best ways is simply to allow yourself to feel hungry before you eat. Every time you eat. When we graze and snack all day we have no relationship with our hunger, which in my book is an essential component to understanding or recognising when we are satiated. Food can never fix whatever issue you are gorging for: chocolate to heal a broken heart, grazing at the fridge door because you are bored, hiding under the duvet with a chunk of Brie to alleviate your sorrow. Food will never cure whatever is eating you.

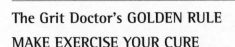

The Grit Doctor's GOLDEN RULE
MAKE EXERCISE YOUR CURE

EXERCISE

Exercise your hunger

I get hungry every four hours or so and tend to eat in four-hourly cycles. You may be different. So to begin with, let yourself go for however long it takes until you recognise that you are hungry, which you will experience as a physical drive to find food (common cues: stomach rumbling, feeling a bit weak, finding it hard to concentrate). This is your cue to eat. Now. Delay eating and you risk a ridiculous binge on all the wrong stuff later on. If you eat when you are hungry your brain is able to tell you when you've had enough and getting good at this simple caveman technique is a brilliant weapon to have in your crap-cutting arsenal.

A GRIT DOCTOR DISTINCTION
Hunger is a physiological need driven by the body, whereas appetite is a psychological desire driven by the brain.

TIPS

- Get into the habit of leaving proper gaps between eating and drinking (anything other than water) and you will soon be back in touch with feeling hungry.
- Notice when you are eating between meals when you're not hungry, and try to identify what is driving you to the Dairy Milk. Recognise that you are not feeding any physical hunger and remind yourself that what you are doing will not satisfy you and can only perpetuate your weight problem. It is a bad habit that you can break. YOU. CAN. BREAK. IT.
- Find other ways to deal with feelings and use those instead of the proverbial bar of chocolate. Distract and divert yourself. Try knitting, painting, reading, gardening. I recommend anything outdoors and well away from an evil vending machine.
- Exercise is a powerful tool to help manage emotional eating AND get you back in touch with true hunger. Use it.
- Don't use emotional eating as your excuse for remaining overweight. You still always have a choice whether or not to put something into your mouth. Own that choice, don't let it own you.

OLLY'S FOOD DIARY: PART 1

July 2013. Olly's vital statistics: 6 ft tall, 15 stone 4 lb carrying most of the excess around his middle. BMI: 29 (30 is classed as obese).[18]

Aiming for a BMI of between 20 and 25, so 13 stone 3 lb or thereabouts. Olly is adamant that any 'thinner' than this would be too thin for him.

THE GRIT DOCTOR SAYS

My mission for my husband: to undo over the course of writing this book nearly twenty years of bad food habits. FOREVER.

Having studied Olly's diet at close quarters for several years now, I know that a few small tweaks will have a dramatic impact over time. Some crappy features of Olly's diet include:

- Crisps, sweets, chocolate – calorie-busting, salt-and-sugar-addled junk
- Pudding after every evening meal

---

18 I know, I know. I am telling you to bin your scales and Olly is getting weighed. But this is the clearest way for me to demonstrate the success (or otherwise!) of what we're doing, so it is a necessary evil for us all to endure in this particular instance. The scales are going to charity when the book is finished, I promise.

- Pastry snacks
- Huge portions
- Coke and other fizzy drinks – sugar-drenched filth disguised as a thirst quencher
- Seconds
- Late-night snacking – he has a particular penchant for popcorn with chocolate pieces mixed in[19]
- Buying snacks from petrol stations on journeys or buying anything other than petrol and water when travelling
- Full-fat lattes

Olly is a criminal barrister, so his daily routine can vary hugely depending on which court he is going to and what stage his trial is at. I know from my own time at the bar that courts are culinary wastelands, offering only heavy 'school dinner' style meals, with the only other option being the vending machine.[20] Anyway, on account of the poor-quality meals (which are also ludicrously expensive) and the lack of proximity to and/or the practicality of getting to a café/supermarket etc. for alternatives during a lunch break (rarely taken), it is very easy to cave in to a sugary hit from the evil vending machine. So it is important to keep his

19 This is also a GD fave, so not to be spurned forever but to be put firmly back into its correct position as a very occasional treat. Remember that it is never the naughty treat or unhealthily delicious snack that is the problem per se, it's the naughty treat's elevation to daily staple that is the real issue.

20 Incidentally, The Grit Doctor would have all such machines banned, particularly in and around schools and wherever else fat kids lurk. BANNED – no less.

sugar levels consistent and avoid his energy levels dipping by preventing him feeling hungry.

I am aiming for an Olly who no longer bulk buys biscuits and chocolates at the supermarket which I then have to hide. Not because he has been banned (entirely futile, as I have tried this tack many times), but because he'll choose other foods. Fresh, nutritious products which he will learn to prefer, or perhaps, more accurately, learn to *value*, once he has experienced the link between what he eats and how he looks and feels fitness-wise. Over time this must *surely* become much more appealing than any short-lived sugar high.

So part of the plan is going to involve a decent breakfast (he always skips breakfast) and organising a packed lunch every day. I anticipate that those two changes alone will make a huge difference to his weight and wellbeing. Olly's list is probably fairly common for many of us, so have a good look at it, and identify where it applies to you. Just crossing off a few things from that list and sticking to them will have a massive impact over time. Please don't go for the whole lot straight off the bat.

THE GRIT DOCTOR WILL SEE YOU NOW

Q: Why can't I change everything NOW?
I am feeling so motivated!

A: Because if you try to change lots of things at once, there will be lots of things you can fail at and too many adjustments for your body and mind to take on, which will have you feeling like you do on a diet: in a state of permanent sacrifice. So, even if it seems too easy, I strongly recommend taking one bad habit at a time and turning it into a Crap-Cutting Commitment.

CRAP-CUTTING COMMITMENTS (CCC)

EXERCISE

Make a CRAP TO CUT list of your own where you identify all your bad eating habits, using Olly's own list on pages 37–38 as a template to help you. Stick it up on the fridge next to your fat photo and allocate each bad habit a month of the year in which you are going to commit to cutting it from your life. For good.

It would be too much for Olly, or anyone with this sort of list of bad habits, to be expected to drop them all at once. A bad habit took a long time to embed, and will take time to break, so once your list is complete, have a good look at it and pick just one of those habits to tackle right now – making it **January's Crap-Cutting Commitment.**

If you are feeling gritty and uber-motivated, capitalise on this feeling and go for a big one – your killer bad habit. Crisps, sweets, chocolate, cake, pastry eating or cola drinking on a daily basis are all killer bad habits. If you are feeling weaker willed, go for one you feel confident you can tackle successfully, like giving up full-fat lattes and going for skinnies instead. If you are faffing around at this stage decorating your list and are at a loss for which one to go for, choose 'having seconds after a meal'. All you need to change eating-wise for the rest of reading this book is to stick to that one commitment. When you succeed – which you will – the confidence generated will help you to tackle the next one, **February's Crap-Cutting Commitment**, until they are all eradicated from your life.

I want you to think of your Crap-Cutting Commitments as individual hurdles which you will tackle *one at a time until nailed*. Something is nailed when it has become a good habit, you don't have to think about it so much any more and are able to do it easily, like brushing your teeth. Once that skinny macchiato is second nature then and only then is it time to embrace your next CCC. Slowly, slowly, catchy monkey. THIS IS FOR THE REST OF YOUR LIFE, so there is no hurry. The more organic you are able to make this feel, the more likely it is to stick and the more effortless it will be to embrace. Which is the polar opposite of dieting: forcing you to feel your sacrifice so keenly that you become utterly obsessed with all those foodstuffs you are denied.

THE GRIT DOCTOR WILL SEE YOU NOW
Q: But Grit Doctor, why a month?

A: A month is basically the Lenten period, which has never failed to work for me to nail a bad habit. I gave up sugar in my coffee for Lent many years ago and couldn't bear the taste of sugar in it thereafter. If you give something up for Lent, it's as good as given up forever. Plus on a practical level, it's easy to remember, and it slows and calms down the process so you are tackling your bad eating habits in doable bite-sized chunks. Which is one of the keys to your success.

PART 2

THE HOLY GRAIL

3

SAPS

Before we can begin to successfully abandon all forms of dieting forever, we need to re-engage with our common sense and accept some basic rules that provide the foundations upon which a healthy lifestyle can be built. Underpinning your individual Crap-Cutting Commitments are these non-negotiable rules.

May I also take this moment to remind you that I am not a nutritionist or dietician, although given their wildly contradictory and conflicting opinions and advice on what's best to eat, this may be to mine and your advantage. The point is I am not here to tell you what precise combination of proteins and carbs is going to magically kick-start the fat-burning process, *because there isn't one.* If there were, there would be just one universal diet *that actually worked* more than three per cent of the time.

What I am trying to get you to do is find a way of being healthier and eating less crap that you are able to implement successfully in your life, for good. You need to adopt an eating regime that works for you. To illustrate this point, a short story about one of my best friends. He lives and dies by the 'never mix proteins with barely-there carbs' method and he does look pretty darn buff on it. He and his partner are both on the same regime and have been for a few years, so it has become a way of life, a way of being healthy that works well for them. Great. They are both at healthy weights and neither reports any ill effects from a high-protein diet. They don't have children. This way of eating wouldn't work for loads of other people, myself included. I exist on the opposite kind of regime: high-carbohydrate foods are the mainstay of my meals and I find they fuel my lifestyle and running perfectly. Neither my friend nor I are trying to lose weight as we are both slim. We both feel good about our food choices and both work out regularly yet we're eating oppositional diets.

The critical point that bears repeating is that you have to do what works *for you*. If you love carbs as I do, and they agree with your body,[21] find ways of making them work for you, but don't

21 The Grit Doctor is gluten-intolerant intolerant. Unless you have a genuine allergy (which can only be confirmed by a real doctor – no self-diagnosis, please) get over it. You may actually be creating the very intolerance you are seeking to avoid by prematurely restricting food groups from your diet. I remember my mum used to say, 'nobody is allergic in my house' – a step too far, perhaps . . . well, it was when my bestie went into anaphylactic shock, JOKE – but there is something in that. It cannot be possible that the number of people who claim to be are *genuinely* gluten and lactose intolerant. Most likely you have become allergic to exercise and might find that a brisk walk would cure you of that 'bloated' feeling of which you so often complain. If you think it makes you sound interesting to talk of your various intolerances and allergies, while spurning the home-made bread that has been lovingly prepared for you, you have gone horribly wrong. Desperately crappy thinking I'm afraid and even crappier chat.

try and cut them out as you will set yourself up for a colossal fail. Carbs themselves have never been the real enemy, nor has any one combination of food groups.

THE GRIT DOCTOR SAYS

We are looking for a healthier way of living and eating that works with *your* body and *your* tastes.

With the above in mind . . .

THE HOLY GRAIL

SUGAR: *Less of this*

ACTIVITY: *More of this*

PROCESSED FOODS: *Fewer of these*

Leads to: **S**ETTLING DOWN WEIGHT

THE GRIT DOCTOR SAYS

SAPS: Aptly named because getting this wrong saps you of your mojo and keeps you trapped in a fatter than necessary body.

Think 'SAPS' when you are choosing food. Is it sugar-loaded? Does it come in plastic and take three minutes to cook in a microwave? Yes? Then choose something else. Have I been sitting on my fat arse all day? Get outside for a walk. Have the word SAPS seared into your brain and think SAPS when choosing and eating food – it is easy to remember, broad in scope and begs the key mindful question: 'Is this food going to GIVE me energy or SAP me of it?'

It *cannot* be this simple, I hear you object. This is too obvious and straightforward. What about chia seeds? Coconut water? Acai? Kale breadless soulless sarnies? Spinach smoothies? Special teas? Red meat? Pasta? Quinoa? Gwyneth Paltrow? Antioxidants? Enzymes? Essential fatty acids? Detox? Weight-loss supplements? Vitamin tablets? Eating carbs after 2 p.m.? Mixing carbs and proteins? Paleo? Organic superfoods? Goji berries? Caffeine? Egg-white omelettes?

Look, you can fanny around with health supplements and superfoods as much as you like; follow fads, get obsessive about coconut water if you so choose and spuff a small fortune on chia seeds. Maybe some of it will impact upon your health and sense of wellbeing for the length of time that the 'craze' lasts or can hold your interest and appetite, but there is no single food-stuff or product that will yield as positive an impact on your quality of life and weight management as taking up regular exercise will.

OLLY'S FOOD DIARY: PART 2

10 September. *He has lost a stone!* Still no sign of a six pack or any abs as yet. Will report as soon as any underlying muscle tone emerges.

Recently on a Saturday I had a terrible craving for pizza and full-fat Coke. I know, I know! Shock. Horror. This is a very rare occurrence, but I just had to have it. Olly used to be a once-a-week Domino's man, but since his healthy eating regime we haven't had a single takeaway. Anyway, we had the pizza and Coke, all at my instigation it has to be said. The next morning Olly complained of feeling really bloated and unhappy about the pizza binge and he promptly offered to take the twins to the park as he said he needed to burn off some of the pizza! *I am in love with this man*. At last he is speaking my language. I knew I would feel bloated and guilty and want to run afterwards. Because running is a normal part of my routine it was no biggie. But Olly had never before complained after eating junk, nor had he ever made any link between what he had eaten and how he was feeling. BINGO. He is becoming much more in tune with his body. He is listening to it, cherishing it and wants to feed it with the good stuff. My work is almost done.

4

FOOD GROUP ESSENTIALS

FRUIT AND VEGETABLES

This food group is your key to successful weight management. Dramatically upping your intake at the expense of the other food groups is a failsafe way to both lose weight *and keep that weight off*. Five portions a day is a bare minimum target but you really want to aim much higher than that. The Japanese and traditional Greek diets are arguably the healthiest in the world and plants have pride of place in their diets.

Don't panic about portion sizes. A piece of fruit is a portion. And a normal amount of vegetables with a meal or a side salad is a portion. A handful of berries is a portion. Whenever in doubt just GO LARGE, as you really can't overdo fruit and veg, no matter what some silly diets will have us believe. As a rule of thumb you want to be getting more of your daily portions from vegetables than fruit, ideally double.

CRAP CONFUSION

Have you heard any of the following?

- Avoid below the ground vegetables e.g. sweet potatoes, beets, turnips, carrots as they are full of sugar, and only eat vegetables that grow above the ground
- Try to stick to fruits that are of the berry variety
- Do not eat bananas and pineapple as they are full of sugar
- Mangoes, cherries, grapes and tangerines must be avoided because of their high fructose content

All of the above is CRAP. Ignore *anything* you hear or read about cutting any form of fresh vegetable or fruit from your diet. The truth is we are just not eating enough. If you are struggling to reach five a day, but would easily meet that target (or better still, beat it) with sweet potato, pineapple and carrots on board then, for the love of God, eat them. It is *always* better to eat a root vegetable or a banana than a packet of crisps or a processed microwave meal. Got it?

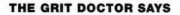

THE GRIT DOCTOR SAYS

If you happen to love mangoes and yams, and would gladly swap them for your chips and ice-cream, great. Make the swap. There is plenty of time for fine-tuning a basically healthy diet later on.

Recipe: Steak night

We have steak probably once a month or every six weeks; we had this last night and it was delicious. I always buy smallish steaks and before cooking trim off the outer layer of fat because otherwise Olly will gobble his, and then mine.[22] There is plenty of fat within the steak marbling to ensure it still has bags of flavour, plus the outer fat shrinks at a different temperature from the meat, resulting in uneven cooking – which is the clever excuse I give Olly for depriving him of it.

PS: I had been on a six-mile run in the rain in the morning. And the quantity of veg was at least five portions' worth each.

You will need (for two people):

---

22 Gobbling bacon rind, lamb and pork chop fat or the fat on your steak can set you back hundreds of calories, so cut it out.

1 bag ready-cubed sweet potato (or 2 sweet potatoes cut into
  chunks)

1 bag trimmed fine green beans

2 bunches trimmed asparagus

2 small steaks – whatever cut is your favourite, ribeye is mine – with
  the outer layer of fat trimmed off

2 large handfuls young spinach leaves, washed

Roast a bag of cubed sweet potato for 30 minutes at 180°C (350°F) fan assisted with a tablespoon of olive oil (I put all the sweet potato into a bowl and use my hands to make sure everything gets a coating of oil. This is a good way of ensuring you always use less. An even better way is to cut your veg in bigger chunks but Olly bought a bag from M&S already in tiny cubes). Turn off the oven and leave them in there to keep warm.

Cook the green beans (3–4 minutes in boiling water) and asparagus (2–3 minutes – I chucked them in with the beans after a minute or so) to *al dente*.

While the veg is cooking, I cook the steaks (with a tablespoon of vegetable oil – in total – rubbed on to both sides of both steaks, seasoned and left to rest at room temperature) by getting the frying pan so hot you can see the smoke coming off it and then chucking them in. Cook for 1 minute on each side for rare and add a small knob of butter at the end, say half a tablespoon's worth.

Transfer the steaks to a plate to rest and into the hot buttery juice in the frying pan (with the heat now off) wilt a couple of big handfuls of young spinach leaves and then chuck in the sweet potato cubes and greens and give everything a coating with the buttery steak juices. Pile everything from the pan on to warmed plates and place the steaks on top.

FRUIT AND VEG MYTHS

I had supper with a friend recently who happens to be over-weight, and he proudly announced that he didn't eat root vegetables or potatoes with his lunch — while chowing down on apple pie with ice-cream *and* cream for dessert. This is so arse-about-face it's a joke. Surely it would be far better to have had the roots or potatoes with lunch — cooked healthily — and skipped the cardiac-arrest-inducing pudding in the evening?

So, while it is of course true that certain vegetables and fruits have more sugars in them than others, worry not at this stage about such distinctions. No one ever became obese from eating too many vegetables that grew under the ground.[23] If you are overweight and have banished certain vegetables and fruits from your and your family's diets, or have got into the habit of avoid-ing them because they are 'too sugary', you have gone horribly wrong. Because if you are overweight, this can only mean that

23 You know very well that chips do not count as vegetables.

you are eating something infinitely crappier that more avid apple munching might have helped you steer clear of. You are trying to run before you can walk. Stop.

THE GRIT DOCTOR'S BOTTOM LINE

Never EVER be put off buying fresh fruit or vegetables because of their sugar content.

TIPS FOR REACHING THAT ELUSIVE FIVE-A-DAY:

- Eat *every* meal with a huge portion of vegetables or a side salad. If you are not in the habit of doing so, this is one of the reasons your meals are unnecessarily calorific and less healthy than they could be. Vegetables should always make up a large part of every meal. Except breakfast. Unless, of course, you love fruit and/or vegetables at breakfast. But don't force yourself into being a fruit-and-yoghurt or mushroom muffin kinda gal at brekkie if it goes against the grain for you – as it does me. But at every other meal, vegetables must feature. *Especially* if you are having shepherd's pie or lasagne or spaghetti Bolognese or a burger or whatever the less healthy meals that happen to be your weekly staples are. You must incorporate a huge salad or greens. Make this a habit.

- Get into the habit of reducing the portion size of the main meal in proportion to the increase in greenery. *Especially* when the main meal is of the burger or Bolognese variety. Let's call it *proportionality.*

- Add bulkier vegetables to salads to make them more filling, interesting and nutritious. Just cook until *al dente* (in a steamer is ideal but fast boiling is fine) and rinse under cold water to retain colour and bite. This is a win-win because not only do the vegetables taste and look better but the faster the cooking, the more nutrients are retained. I add green beans and peas to dressed lettuce to have with pasta. Chuck in some chopped fresh herbs too – parsley works in almost everything and is fantastically nutritious, but I often use mint in summer salads, basil if there are tomatoes involved and coriander if I want an Asian flavour. Add some mixed seeds and suddenly your salad has got real personality as well as packing a banging nutritional punch.

- If you are in the habit of snacking and are not yet ready or willing to make quitting it a CCC, snack on raw veg. I love raw peppers at the moment, but carrots and cucumber go with everything, particularly a delicious home-made veggie dip. Having crudités and a dip on hand in the fridge will have you bumping up your veg quota no end, and hopefully will help you stay away from less healthy alternatives.

- Take a piece of fruit everywhere. Or two. An apple, a banana – whatever you like and is easiest on your handbag or rucksack (peaches are not a portable fruit, sadly, and are the enemy of any bag). This is one of the greatest damage limitation exercises you can effortlessly implement in your life.

THE GRIT DOCTOR WILL SEE YOU NOW

Q: What on earth are you talking about damage limitation exercises?

A: Not the peach. But that thing that happens when you sleepwalk into Greggs for a sausage roll when you are feeling a bit peckish at 4 p.m., or mindlessly buy a Twix with your copy of *The Times*. When it comes to the whole five-a-day thing, we are often advised by nutritionists, dieticians and the NHS to keep a piece of fruit about our person, but we continue to ignore this brilliantly simple and effective tip and then fail to understand why we are still nipping into the newsagents at the same time every day for a packet of chocolate buttons.

I have a very veg-heavy lunch every day. Actually, most days it's a veg-only lunch unless I have a sandwich with the twins, which happens a few times a week. I usually manage to get about four veg portions in at lunch and I make sure I have a vegetable protein too because I know from experience that it keeps me feeling full until tea-time. More often than not I choose something of the bean variety; lentil salads, soya bean pasta, that kind of thing. My sweet potato salad (see recipe on page 62), warm with puy lentils stirred through makes a delicious and filling lunch. Aim to eat twice as many vegetable portions as fruit portions as a general rule of thumb.

THE GRIT DOCTOR SAYS

Five a day is the absolute bare minimum. Aim high; go for double that as I do and you will find weight management gets easier with every extra portion you add in.

SALAD MISHAPS

1. Never add sugar to dressings. It's wholly unnecessary. Three parts oil to two parts vinegar and a teaspoon of Dijon mustard is a classic and you can't really go wrong with it. The best quality virgin olive oil you can afford is always what the gurus recommend and is most certainly the healthiest option, but I am not averse to a vegetable oil dressing on occasion. Whichever oil or fat you choose to use, do not pour it freehand over salads. Measure out your oils and fats religiously. Always use less than you think you need and mix

into your leaves/veg with your (impeccably clean) hands so everything gets touched by the dressing. Dress just before eating. If you can't resist grazing after you have finished your meal, graze on what's left in the salad bowl. It really cannot be kept in the fridge so will only go to waste if you don't.

2. Salads become crappy the instant you throw a bottle of Caesar-style dressing or any other creamy/cheesy/ supermarket-bought dressing over them. Make like the Greeks and try to stick to a basic dressing of oil and vinegar or oil and lemon juice. The more effort you make with the salad itself, the less you need to rely on dressing to sex it up. The dressing should never be the main event, and if you can still see any at the bottom of the bowl when the salad is finished you have used too much. Far too much.

3. Salads are a great place to experiment for those a bit shy of cooking up a storm in the kitchen, because it is only really a matter of assembling ingredients, without having to rely on any real technique or culinary skill. Nuts (the fatties among you should be sparing, please), seeds and avocados are fantastic ways to get proteins and healthy unsaturated fats into your salads, not to mention adding taste, colour and texture.

SOME CRAP FREE VEG-FULL SALAD IDEAS

Recipe: Soya bean salad

Cook frozen soya beans according to instructions (as many as you want to make a salad for supper with enough left over to use the next day in a lunchbox). Rinse under cold water to cool and retain the green colour and texture.

For the dressing (enough for 500g cooked soya beans):

A tablespoon of olive oil or sesame oil
Generous squeeze or two of lemon or lime
Pinch of dried chilli flakes
Seasoning to taste

Add the dressing to the soya beans. This salad is lovely on its own, or you can boil some pasta, quinoa or bulgar wheat and stir that through it when cool, adding chopped cherry tomatoes, spring onions and lamb's lettuce, or whatever salad you've got and like – all of which makes for delicious lunchbox material. Experiment with adding fresh herbs: corriander and parsley work very well.

It's great to leave a bowl of soya beans in the fridge for snacking on at the kids' tea-time, to see you through till supper. Or for when you get back from work and just have to nibble on something before you prepare your evening meal.

Recipe: Butternut and Spinach salad (for 4)

A butternut squash, skin on, cut into large chunks, seasoned and
coated in 1 tablespoon of olive oil (use hands)

1 bag young spinach leaves

Large handful fresh basil leaves

Small handful mixed seeds

Juice of half a lemon

Puy lentils (optional extra, cooked according to packet instructions)

Roast butternut at 180°C (350°F) for 30 minutes or until golden, turn off the oven and leave there. Into your serving dish put a tablespoon of olive oil and the lemon juice and to that add the young spinach leaves, whole basil leaves and a handful of mixed seeds (if you can be arsed, they are even better dry fried first). Season to taste. Mix everything together gently with a large spoon, the butternut squash still warm or at room temperature.

We had this salad tonight piled high with grilled mackerel fillets on top and a lemon wedge. We often serve this at barbecues, too. It's colourful and flavourful and more interesting than your bog-standard potatoes and salad. Plus there is minimal work involved: no peeling, barely any chopping or mess and it can be assembled in seconds.

Lentils worked very well as an extra ingredient to add to the leftovers for Olly's lunchbox the following day – which he happily claimed kept him feeling satisfied all afternoon.

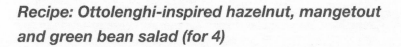

Recipe: Ottolenghi-inspired hazelnut, mangetout and green bean salad (for 4)

Yotam Ottolenghi was and is a huge inspiration to me ever since my husband bought me a cookery lesson with him the first Christmas we were boyfriend and girlfriend. To be honest, at the time I was mortally offended getting sent off for a cooking lesson, *and* it was a cake-making session (my God he is selfish) but the man himself – Ottolenghi that is – was amazing and I just love his vegetable dishes. All of his food, in fact. It was his mangetout and green bean salad that got me making salads with loads of cooked and cold green veg in them and generally inspired a shift towards more exciting vegetable making. The only problem was that before we had kids, I was happy and willing to devote entire days to some of his more complex recipes including the sourcing of obscure ingredients, but now I have to be more time-savvy. But the mangetout and bean salad is a cinch to prepare.

1 small packet of hazelnuts (but other nuts work well)

3 tablespoons olive oil

Zest of 1 orange very finely chopped, avoiding too much bitter white pith

2 garlic cloves, peeled and crushed

Handful of chives, finely chopped (I use scissors to cut chives)

2 bags mangetout

2 bags trimmed extra fine green beans

Dry-roast the hazelnuts for 10 minutes at 180°C (350°F) until golden brown. Remove and bash in a sandwich bag or clean tea towel so some are broken and some are left whole.

For the dressing, mix the olive oil, orange zest (a zester is a really handy thing to have), crushed garlic and chives. Steam or cook the green beans for 2–3 minutes in boiling water, then throw in the mangetout and cook for another 1.5 minutes until everything is *al dente*, then rinse under the cold tap, dry with kitchen paper or a clean tea towel and set aside. When you are ready to serve, just add the dressing to the bottom of your serving bowl and gently mix in the vegetables and top with the nuts.

This salad can be prepared earlier and dressed just before serving, which is ideal for parties. I have also made infinite incarnations – broccoli instead of green beans, asparagus and peas with mixed green leaves, or rocket and watercress often leaving out the orange zest, or no nuts but a handful of mixed seeds instead. You get my drift. The key is the zesty, garlicky dressing, a bit of nutty/seedy texture and the deep green colour of the veg. Experiment.

Recipe: Raw courgette and broad bean salad (for 4)

250g fresh broad beans

2 courgettes cut into long strips (I use a vegetable peeler – cut off
　　both ends of the courgette and peel the whole length to get long,
　　wide and very delicate ribbons)

Handful of fresh mint leaves and flat leaf parsley, finely chopped

2 tablespoons olive oil

Juice of half a lemon

Seasoning

Small handful of crushed walnuts

50g feta cheese

Remove the broad beans from their pods, cook for 3–4 minutes and then de-pod again to reveal the bright green bean underneath. (I have not made this since having children due to the time-consuming nature of the twice-podded broad bean so this recipe is best for the childless. Or those with children old enough to help with the de-podding. Or cheat and use soya beans.) Then add to the raw courgette along with the fresh mint, parsley, olive oil, lemon juice, seasoning and crumbled feta cheese. Scatter the crushed walnuts on top to finish.

Courgettes on their own dressed this way are delicious and make a great accompaniment to any pasta dish.

Recipe: Aubergine and yoghurt with cumin

1 pack baby aubergines

2 or 3 large cloves garlic, sliced very thinly

1–2 tablespoons olive oil

Seasoning

100g full-fat Greek yoghurt

Ground cumin

A pinch of cumin seeds

Slice the aubergines in half lengthways, score the cut surface and brush with olive oil (I find using a brush helps reduce the amount of oil added, as aubergine is to oil what a slice of white toast is to butter: a sponge). Put the sliced garlic into the cuts in the aubergine and sprinkle with some cumin seeds, season well and roast for 30 minutes at 180°C (350°F) or until soft and golden. Once cooked, allow them to cool down to just warm then place a dollop of Greek yoghurt and a small pinch of cumin powder on top of each aubergine half (let the yoghurt reach room temperature first).

I made this recently with roast lamb, left out the olive oil, and instead cooked the aubergines, scored sides down, in the roasting tin where they took on all the lamb juices. Delicious.

Recipe: Roger's chickpea salad recipe (for 4)

300ml/10fl oz natural yoghurt (preferably Greek)

Pinch of salt

Ground pepper

1 tablespoon peeled and finely chopped red onion or spring onion

Approx. 6 oz cooked chickpeas (tinned are fine, but be sure to rinse with cold water and pat dry)

6 cherry tomatoes cut into quarters

½ a cucumber, deseeded and cut into small chunks

1 tablespoon chopped fresh mint (or coriander if preferred)

1 small pinch of cayenne pepper

Lightly beat the yoghurt in a bowl and add all other ingredients. Stir well. Taste and adjust seasoning to your liking. This salad was delicious alongside a green salad and barbecued lamb chops.

TIPS TO VEG UP

- Get out of the bad habit of thinking that unless there is a hunk of meat on your plate, it isn't a proper meal.
- You can make your own 'vegetable hummus' dips so easily and cheaply by just boiling your veg and blitzing (don't be tempted to overboil so it's really mushy as you'll lose nutrients). You do need a blender for this but a hand-held soup one does the trick for me – less washing-up than a full-on Magimix affair. Frozen broad beans (no need to pod here), peas, or peas and soya beans whizzed up with a dollop of Greek yoghurt and mint work brilliantly. You can add olive oil, or feta cheese if you want a richer hummus – although if you're really trying to shift the pounds I'd suggest steering clear at this stage.
- I made a beetroot tsatziki when on holiday in Scotland recently by peeling and grating fresh beets and mixing with full-fat natural yoghurt, one crushed fresh garlic clove, the juice of a lemon, and

some fresh parsley and mint, finely chopped. It was delicious on baps with a slice of ham and made a perfect dip with crudités.

- Vegetarian pasta or risotto meals. Incorporating at least one vegetarian pasta/risotto meal each week is easy, economical and quick – a simple way to veg up, especially when you have your salad or greens accompanying it. I had a fennel risotto recently with a mountain of thin green beans (cooked and then allowed to cool) tossed in a tablespoon of olive oil, a squeeze of lemon and some finely chopped mint. (As I write this, summer is fast approaching and I am managing to grow some mint in the garden, so it's getting chucked into everything.)
- Garlic, chilli flakes/powder, lemon juice and fresh herbs all work brilliantly at jazzing your hummus up a bit without adding calories.

My friend Zoe makes an amazing healthy slaw inspired by London's Pitt Cue Co, which I've adapted here:

Serves 4–6

¾ of a small white cabbage

1 fennel bulb

1 red onion

Handful of fresh mint

Big handful fresh parsley and coriander

Seasoning

Handful of mixed seeds, including fennel seeds

For the dressing:

    3 tablespoons cider vinegar

    3 tablespoons white wine vinegar

    3 tablespoons extra virgin olive oil

1 tablespoon of runny honey

Juice of a lemon

2 tablespoons Greek yoghurt

Put the dressing ingredients into a bowl and whisk together. Set aside.

Slice the cabbage, fennel and onion 1mm thick (on a mandolin if you have one) – the thinner the better – and put it all into a large bowl. Finely chop the herbs and add making sure they are spread evenly throughout the slaw by stirring gently with a large spoon. Chuck in the seeds.

Half an hour before serving, whisk the dressing again, and pour over the slaw. Toss thoroughly and check for seasoning.

This keeps overnight and worked brilliantly the next day for Olly's lunchbox with cold roast chicken.

ALL HAIL KALE?

Kale crisps – a misnomer of the highest order. I'm not sure where there is a place for kale on God's earth, but it is most definitely not in a crisp packet. Kale juice? Honestly, I'd rather neck a litre of absinthe.[24] These days there's always one particular 'superfood' that's in vogue: blueberries, acai berries, chia seeds. 'Scientists' would have us believe that adding these fashionable fruit and veg to our food will immediately turn us into Gwyneth Paltrow. Thank God, they don't.

THE GRIT DOCTOR SAYS

Don't force yourself to like or eat kale. It isn't going to cure you of anything or make you thin. It may make you desperately unhappy as you wonder why, despite its seemingly infinite incarnations, eating it still leaves you feeling suicidal.

Look, I am well aware of kale's position as a superveg, and certainly don't want to put you off it if you love it. What I am trying to do is illustrate that it is far better to work with good foods you actually enjoy eating, than force yourself to consume ones you think you should. This also gets you out of the bad habit of buying whatever food stuff is currently being hailed as the salvation from all our ills.

The point is to experiment and sex up those veggies.

---

24 Confession: I did eat a rather good kale dish recently. Simply whack a large bag of chopped kale onto a baking tray, drizzle with soy sauce, sprinkle with black pepper and roast for 10 minutes at 200°C.

GRIT DOCTOR FRUIT DISTINCTIONS

Dried fruits are fine as an *occasional* snack but they can have a much higher sugar content, unless you are eating them piece for piece, i.e. one slice of dried pineapple has the same sugar content as one slice of the fresh stuff. But there is less sugar in a cup of grapes than there is in a cup of raisins. Got it? Plus, some branded dried fruits have got the nasty High Fructose Corn Syrup added – more of this bad boy later. It goes without saying, though, that dried fruit (HFCS-infused crap excepted) is infinitely preferable to a biscuit/cake/sweets/sausage roll aberration.

THE GRIT DOCTOR SAYS

You are going to want sugar at some stage every day. Choose the naturally occurring sugar in fresh fruit and vegetables 80 per cent of the time and you've got your sugars nailed.

Freshly frozen vegetables and fruits really help to keep you on top of your five-a-day by providing a brilliant standby when the fresh stuff has run out and acting as a much cheaper and readily available alternative to fresh without sacrificing any nutritional value. We all eat frozen peas but we're not so good at stocking up on frozen broccoli, cauliflower (already cut into perfect florets for gratins, bakes and the like) and frozen spinach (in dense handy portions). My kids won't eat cooked spinach on its own (although I recently discovered they do like the raw young leaves) but it gets whizzed into the passata that becomes their pasta sauce and they never complain. I add frozen berries to huge fruit salads too. This saves on cost, obviously, but on hassle too, as there is no washing, peeling or faffing involved – just chuck the bag in.

THE GRIT DOCTOR WARNS

Do not try to source any of your five-a-day from drinks. Drinks don't count.

Ruth

I sex up a fruit salad by grating fresh ginger and orange zest into the juice of one or two oranges and a tablespoon of finely chopped fresh mint (if I've got any knocking about) into a large bowl. I leave this in the bottom of the bowl, then start adding all the fruits. Mix them up gently with a spoon and serve with a big dollop of full-fat Greek yoghurt on top.

GRIT DOCTOR RESEARCH

In its December 2013 edition, the *British Medical Journal* claimed that if an apple a day was prescribed to all adults aged fifty and over, 8,500 vascular deaths such as heart attacks and strokes would be prevented or delayed each year in the UK.

An apple a day is The Grit Doctor Way.

STARCHY FOODS

Aka *carbs*, these are what we need for energy and they form the baseline of my family's meals. Wholemeal bread, wholegrain rice and cereals are miles better for you than their refined counterparts. I find wholewheat pasta a step too far as I love the white stuff too much to make the sacrifice. This is fine. We are not aiming for perfection, just a less crappy diet than the one we are currently enjoying. I love wholegrain breads and I genuinely prefer brown rice to white because of its nutty flavour. Those brown carbs are also a great source of fibre – vital for keeping everything moving through our guts but lacking from most of our diets. Try to keep on skins and husks where you can. Baked potatoes, roasted (unpeeled) carrots, sweet potatoes and butternut squash in their skins and wholegrain rice with husks are all fantastically fibrous.

Since writing this book we have started eating bulgar wheat and quinoa (often mixed together) and pearl barley (which I learned on holiday makes for a fantastic rice replacement in risotto) as white rice and potato substitutes. And the twins love all of them. Faff-free, too, as there's no peeling and chopping involved. Plus, they keep in the fridge much better than cooked spuds and make excellent lunchbox material the next day mixed with vegetables and/or salads. Don't get your knickers in a twist about whether you should stop eating grains, as many popular diets currently suggest. I would die were I made to go a single day without my beloved carbs.

THE GRIT DOCTOR SAYS

If you lean towards the carby side of the food spectrum, fruit and vegetables alone are not going to satisfy you, especially when you factor in the *A* part of *SAPS*. The key is to make sure you get your carbs from the best places: GO WHOLEFOOD[25] AND GO BROWN.

CARB CRAP-CUTTING

- If – sorry, *when* – like me, you have a very active lifestyle, and providing you don't have any genuine allergies/issues with

---

25 More a product of nature than a product of industry.

gluten, you can, for the most part, devour carbs without guilt.
But there is no doubt that refined carbs do not provide as high
quality a fuel as their more complex sisters. So try and get most
of your starchy carbs from low GI sources.[26] Low GI is the way
forward because such carbs release their energy slowly, keeping
you fuller for longer and your insulin levels from falling off the
national grid. Because all carbohydrates break down into sugar,
you want those sugars coming at you in a slow, steady stream to
avoid any dramatic dips which can result in a desperate sprint to
the cake shop: keeping your sugar levels consistent is one of the
keys to successful weight maintenance, no question.

- Cereals. Obviously you know that crappy ones like Coco Pops
and Frosties need to be avoided (you may as well spoon white
sugar into the mouths of your children before sending them off
to school). But it's the deceptively 'healthy' ones like Special K
and Shreddies, which I was happily giving the twins until I
discovered they contain more sugar (6.8 and 6.2 grams
respectively) than a slice of McVitie's chocolate cake (5.4g), that
you need to watch. Worthy granola-type cereals are equally
deceptive. If you think about it, granola is essentially grains
knitted together with liquid sugar. Muesli also varies wildly on
the crap scale. Alpen, for example, is made up of 23% sugar;

26 The glycaemic index (GI) estimates how much each gram of available carbohydrate in
a food raises a person's blood glucose level following consumption of the food, relative to
consumption of pure glucose.

Dorset Cereals Simply Delicious Muesli: 16.8% sugar.[27] Much safer to mix up your own muesli using wholefood ingredients if you really love the stuff. Otherwise, stick to Weetabix, Shredded Wheat, oatmeal or oatbran. And be rigorous about checking labels, no matter how worthy the packaging. Don't be deceived by the low-calorie content of what the label describes as a 'portion' – often just 30g which is the equivalent of a measly 3 or 4 tablespoons. What sort of teenager is satisfied on that, I wonder? This of course only matters if cereal is your thang. Worry not at all if it isn't. There are infinitely better, less processed options for breakfast. I can no longer stomach cereal since reading a savage article about it being cattle feed and not fit for human consumption and so stick to wholemeal toast.

CRAP-CUTTING COMMANDMENT
Go brown. Go wholefood.

THE GRIT DOCTOR WILL SEE YOU NOW
Q: How can I tell which are low GI carbs?

A: Don't get bogged down in all this. After all, vegetables and fruits are carbohydrates, and the

---

27 All gleaned from painstaking Grit Doctor research scouring labels in Sainsbury's and my kitchen cupboards.

crap-cutting way is to eat more of ALL vegetables and fruit, irrespective of their GI rating. More often than not, brown wholefoods are low GI. So to that end, find the brownest alternative to your beloved white bread/rice/pasta and, if you like it, stick to it most of the time. We have learned to love the seediest nuttiest brownest of breads at home, but that's not to say that we don't also love a French stick occasionally. And white rice is always better than deep-fried chips. Got it?!

PROTEINS

Proteins (meat, fish, eggs and beans) are essential for growth and repair of the body. Eating them with your carbs is a very good idea because they keep you fuller for longer.

Ruth

This is where a lot of people are going wrong. My dad said to me over Easter, 'I just had two pork chops and a salad for lunch – no potatoes or bread.' Well bloody done. This is just picking and choosing bits of now-outmoded diets at random – Atkins, Beach, Zone, for example – and thinking that mixing carbs with proteins at the same meal somehow makes you fat and that if you don't eat them together you will miraculously lose weight. It doesn't work like that as a one-off. It does if you are ruthless about it, and can bring about ketosis.[28] Far better to have had a much smaller pork chop, a baked potato and a bigger salad with that meal with an eye to his overall calorie intake rather than his carb/protein ratios. Why? Because it is a much more realistic and sustainable way to approach weight management. Unless you follow a high-protein diet religiously (and sometimes at the expense of your health), what you may end up doing is eating a high-fat, high-calorie diet instead. Much better to try and develop a better way of eating that you can actually stick to forever. I don't think about ratios at mealtimes or mixing carbs with proteins; instead I look at a plate and check to make sure it's got loads of green veg on it and isn't swimming in fat.

PROTEIN POINTERS

- The more you can source your proteins from plants, the better. The soya bean is a complete protein[29] and one of the reasons why the Japanese diet is one of the healthiest in the world.

---

28 Defined as a condition characterised by raised levels of ketone in the body, associated with abnormal fat metabolism and diabetes mellitus. GD translation: ketosis is what happens when the body, starved of carbs, has to resort to burning fat for energy instead.

29 A 'complete protein' is one that contains all the essential amino acids. Most plants and vegetables only contain some, whereas meats and fish have the lot. So the soya bean is well worth making friends with, particularly if you are a vegetarian.

- Fish is also a superior protein source to meat if you are weight-watching as it is infinitely lower in fat and calories. Oily fish is also a rich source of omega-3 fatty acids which is fantastic brain food – *chows down on mackerel salad while devising the eating plan that will change the world*. Eat fish at least twice a week – more if you love it. Canned and smoked varieties are cheap and convenient but can be super salty so be aware of this. Tinned mackerel, sardines or tuna on a toasted bagel or wholemeal toast is great for a healthy fast-food emergency meal. Wherever possible buy fish in spring water rather than brine or oil. If you are using fish in oil or brine, make sure you drain the fish thoroughly to minimise the calorie damage, and scour the labels for junk before buying from supermarkets. We have started ordering our fish in bulk from Cornwall, following the lead from friends of ours. So the freezer gets stocked full of mackerel, sea bass, cod and prawns and we make a massive saving as we are getting wholesale prices. We have no excuse not to have at least two or three fish suppers a week, and it spares us the agony of embarrassing ourselves in the fishmongers with our lack of knowledge and panic-fuelled orders.
- Eggs and pulses, beans, nuts and seeds are also great sources of protein. Nuts are high in fibre and a good alternative to snacks high in saturated fat (e.g. crisps or anything resembling them – not that you will be touching one again after doing the exercise on page 168). Almonds are fantastically nutritious and my nut of choice. It's true that nuts are very fatty, so it's best to

eat them in moderation, but if you are going to get your fats in (as you must) they don't come much higher grade than this. Seeds are much lower in calories so wade into them with gusto.

- Trim all obvious fat from meat. And make this a habit. Go for leaner white meats where possible. Chop meat up more often (rather than routinely serving it as one slab) and incorporate into a stew or stir-fry or curry. Makes meat go a lot further, it's kind on the purse, and kinder on the waistline.

- Red meat needs to be downgraded to 'occasional treat' status. If you can give it up completely, go ahead. I'm afraid I love it too much and so does my husband, but we have massively cut down and it is no longer a daily, or even weekly, staple.

- Cutting out red meat as a main source of protein is a crap-cutting essential – not because it is bad *per se*, but because it forms the mainstay of many convenience foods: pies, sausage rolls, burgers, frozen lasagnes and the like. More on this later.

THE GRIT DOCTOR ADVISES

Seeds for you fatties, nuts for you skinnies. And all nuts cease to be healthy foods once coated in salt or honey.

Ruth

I bought a mixed seed carton (linseeds, sesame, sunflower, pumpkin, poppy seeds) from M&S ages ago and buy separate bags of those seeds from Sainsbury's to top up the handy-sized carton; you can easily make up your own mix and just shove it in a jam jar. I leave it out by the salt and pepper and olive oil to try and remember to add those seeds wherever they might work in stews, salads, vegetable bakes etc.

EXERCISE

Put yourself off red meat

Close your eyes and ask yourself: how can I be absolutely sure that this frozen meatball is not in fact horse or dog meat or ammonia-rinsed meat filler that can actually cause cancer?[30] Bring to mind herds of cattle reared for beefburgers penned in so tightly that they give each other skin sores and can barely breathe. Recall the recent horsemeat-in-ready-meals scandal: Think horse and *just. Say. NAY.*

CRAP-CUTTING COMMANDMENT

Dramatically reduce your consumption of cheap red meat. Good quality red meat costs the earth so if you are buying a beefburger for a quid, you can be quite sure it ain't made of beef.

---

30 Jamie Oliver recently won a campaign that had McDonald's reveal all the crap that actually goes into its 'beef' patties and pledge to do better.

MILK AND DAIRY FOODS

Cheese and yoghurt are good sources of protein. And of course they also contain calcium, which helps to keep your bones healthy. Really *essential* for the kids but not ideal for weight watchers, so an area over which to be particularly mindful.

DAIRY DO-GOODERS

- Cottage cheese is a great product to introduce into the fridge. It's low in fat, high in protein and it adds creaminess and texture to dishes without adding many calories. It's also a great snack to dip crudités in.

- Make friends with skimmed milk, or at the very least, semi-skimmed – especially if you drink a lot of cappuccinos and eat cereals because the saving in calories is well worth it. In a typical cappuccino prepared using non-fat milk, there are about 11 grams of carbohydrates, 9 of them that are sugar (but don't panic, it is just sugar that naturally occurs in the milk), 7 grams of protein and 0 grams of fat. Fail to ask for the skinny option, though, and you will end up with the whole milk variety, which contains 6 grams of fat, 4 of which are artery-clogging saturated fat.[31] Plus it will set you back hundreds of calories. All washed

31 We are aiming for just 20g of saturated fat per day for women and 30g for men according to NHS guidelines.

down mindlessly on the way to work. And that's just the first one of the morning: repeat a couple of times a day and those fats and calories really add up.

THE GRIT DOCTOR REASSURES

The taste difference is minimal once you make like a Catholic and swap to non-fat for Lent. Trust me, you will never look back.

Recipe: Cottage cheese pasta

Sounds revolting to anyone who has bad memories of cottage cheese being horrid, tasteless diet food, but this is delicious and makes for great lunchbox leftovers too.

For 2, all you need is:

1 punnet of cherry tomatoes, halved and seasoned
Large handful of fresh basil leaves, torn
Half a large carton of cottage cheese or a whole small one
3 tablespoons olive oil

Simply boil whatever pasta you fancy until *al dente* and then chuck in all the other ingredients and season to taste. Serve immediately.

This is lovely warm and is also delicious cold. I chucked in some leftover soya beans from the salad I'd made earlier (see recipe on page 61) for next day's lunchbox for Olly, which made a colourful change from the night before and beefed up the protein while remaining plant-based. Super healthy.

FAT AND SUGAR

Most people in the UK eat too much fat and too much sugar, so it is this fifth and final food group which is the real problem area. And it's a massive problem, because although fat and sugar really ought to just be the icing on the cake of our diets, for many of us they have become the entire sponge. Saturated fats have long been considered the dietary bad boys, raising cholesterol and increasing our risk of heart disease – but this is currently the subject of argument.[32] Given that it wasn't long ago that margarine was considered to be our saviour from the 'evil' saturated fat found in butter, but is now universally acknowledged to be pure filth, it's hardly surprising that we feel sceptical about everything we read when it comes to sugar and fats.

32 Aseem Malhotra, a leading cardiologist, claims in a recent *British Medical Journal* that it isn't saturated fats themselves that are the problem: milk, cheese and red meat are all good he argues, it's the processed varieties bringing very little nutritional benefit that are the killers.

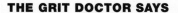

THE GRIT DOCTOR SAYS

Our over-consumption of the saturated fats found in
cakes, pies, junk foods, frozen foods, biscuits and
supermarket pizzas – to name but a few of our
favourites – are no doubt a big contributor to
'problem obesity'.

Unsaturated fats, thankfully, provide the antidote, giving us the
essential fatty acids we need to help us stay healthy, while lowering cholesterol. Oily fish, nuts and seeds, avocados, olive oils
and vegetable oils are great sources and are unarguably healthy.
And, surprise surprise, the Greeks – who have a much lower rate
of heart disease – also have a diet rich in olive oil, fish, nuts, vegetables and salads.

GRIT DOCTOR COMMANDMENT

Eat like the Greeks.

Recipe: Greek salad

Greek salad is a staple in our house. We love feta cheese and love
holidaying in Greece where we eat this by the bucketload. Find

the best freshest tomatoes and the finest olives and olive oil you can source. With the tomatoes it doesn't really matter what sort you use although I like beef tomatoes, but the real key is the freshness and quality of all the ingredients.

For 4, you will need:

4 or 5 beef tomatoes

1 medium red onion, peeled

1 cucumber

1 green pepper

Handful each of fresh parsley, dill and/or mint

1 large handful top notch olives, green or black or both, stoned

1 tablespoon red wine vinegar

3 tablespoons good-quality Greek extra virgin olive oil

A block of feta cheese

1 teaspoon dried oregano

Seasoning

At the bottom of your large salad bowl carefully measure and pour the olive oil and red wine vinegar. Add a pinch of sea salt and some pepper. Finely dice the red onion, then cut the tomatoes into big chunks and place both the onion and tomato in the bowl. Cut the cucumber into thick half-moons, de-seed, then cut the pepper into small chunks and place it all in the salad bowl. Mix gently with a large spoon to dress ingredients, then add your herbs, finely chopped, and the olives. Crumble up the whole block of feta, sprinkle it with the dried oregano and chuck it on top just before you serve up.

A great tip from Jamie Oliver – blitz the leftovers with a few ice cubes and another tablespoon of olive oil to make a Greek gazpacho. Serve in small long water glasses as a starter at a summer lunch barbecue to be enjoyed while standing around in the garden watching the fire burn . . .

EXERCISE

So there are good fats and bad fats, and some of the good fats turned out to be bad fats after all and some of the bad fats may in fact be good fats. With all this in mind, let's simplify matters.

FATS TEST

- Pork pie
- Unsalted almonds
- Avocado
- Sausage roll
- Sunflower seeds
- Scotch egg

Looking at that list, which do you think contain the good fats and which are the bad boys? The key is not to overthink it. One of the problems with modern-day diets is that we have over-complicated food to such a profound extent that we have blinded ourselves to the bleeding obvious. Back to basics please.

TRANS FATS

Trans fats are the crappiest of all – unnatural, man-made, created in factory vats and close cousins to plastic, they crop up in your low-fat margarines, diet spreads, baked goods and processed ready meals. Consider them to be filth and treat them with the same disdain a faeces-eating fly does. Because even flies turn their noses up at trans fats.

EXERCISE

Gritty exercise to put you off trans fats

Never use margarine as a substitute for butter. It is but one molecule away from being plastic. Margarine and diet spreads have *no place* in your kitchen – let alone in your digestive tract, which cannot break them down. Margarine is chock full of trans fats, which have been linked to weight gain, cancer, diabetes and heart disease. So here's a quick exercise: put a tub of margarine in your garden and leave it there. (If you don't have a garden or balcony, just put the margarine tub on your windowsill.) It will not 'go off', it will not grow mould and it will remain untouched – even by insects. Gaze upon the filthy, virtually-plastic gunk and remind yourself that this substance, which you have been spreading on your bread, is not real food. Your body cannot break down and digest plastic (instead it wraps it in fat and stores it in your body) so eating so-called 'slimming' spreads and 'diet' foods can make you fatter even when the calories are deceptively low because it ain't real food and so your body doesn't know what to do with it.

Hopefully this exercise will repel you from this crap for ever-more.[33]

THE GRIT DOCTOR SAYS

The safest way to trim dodgy fats from your diet is to cut out processed foods and go unsaturated wherever you can.

BE FAT WISE

I was struck while watching *Secret Eaters* last night (*ahem* research, my dears) how many calories were wasted in a diet where the bottle of olive oil was wielded too liberally. Thousands

33 Marisa Peer *You Can Be Thin*

of calories being chucked needlessly about salads and meats and potatoes, which turn potentially healthy food into junk and are a serious enemy to your waistline. Any oil, no matter how healthy its press, is still pure fat – olive oil being no exception. Butter, of course, is the same.

Be mindful when you add it to stuff and try to trim it down wherever possible. If you have half-melted chunks of butter on your toast, you have massively overdone it. Never use cold butter from the fridge to make sandwiches or to spread on toast as you will always use at least double what you need. Spread it super thinly and get anal about this, always striving to use less. It is full of flavour and you can still really taste it even when you are using a mere smidgen of the stuff. The same applies to baked potatoes too – a healthy, cheap, fibreful food is turned into junk by adding half a pound of butter. Try a teaspoon of butter and a dollop of cottage cheese or yoghurt and mash it all in, creaming those potato insides up nicely.

THREE SIMPLE AND EFFECTIVE FAT-WISE TIPS:

1. Trim all excess fat and skin from meat before cooking.
2. Always pour your oils on to a spoon first to measure. It gets you into the habit of becoming more mindful of how much you are adding. Bear in mind that a tablespoon of olive oil or vegetable oil contains a whopping 120 calories, all pure fat. You never need that much oil to cook with, particularly extra

virgin olive oil which has a deliciously strong flavour. I'd much rather pour a teaspoon of the raw stuff over my food once it's cooked to get all of the health benefits and the best flavour from it. Same with butter. Start with just a teaspoon of the stuff and add more in teaspoon by teaspoon. If you routinely take a knife to the butter slab and chuck it in and can see butter at the bottom of your pan when you remove the meat or fish or whatever you're cooking, or there is always a layer of oil swimming on the top of your sauces, you may as well decorate your casserole with a bumper packet of KitKats.

3. Never keep cream – single or double – in the fridge. If you do you will find yourself adding it to everything and with every spoonful, a needless extra 70 calories goes into your food. Try Greek yoghurt instead.

SUGAR

Sugar occurs naturally in many foods, including fruit, vegetables and milk, and as you know, all carbohydrates are broken down into sugar by the body. But it is not these types of sugar that we need to worry about, despite what the latest food fad may say. Diets that instruct you to cut out all sugar from your diet are full of crap and part of the reason you are failing. More on this hot topic later.

CRAP-CUTTING COMMANDMENT

However, if you are overweight, fat and sugar is your problem area – guaranteed. So, listen up. If you don't think you eat too much sugar or saturated fat because sweets, chocolate bars or pork pies are not your thing, but you are fat, *you have been fooled.* Pay very close attention to the next section.

EXERCISE

Food diary

A lot of us are very defensive about our diets and delude ourselves that we are eating far more healthily than we actually are. I surprised myself when I tried out this exercise and discovered that I too was doing this.

If you are overweight (and don't want to be) or you're a crappy eater (and don't want to be) and can't work out where you are going wrong, keep a food diary for a week. It doesn't matter how you do it – scribble things down in a notebook, or use an actual diary to write in. Take it with you everywhere and record every morsel and drink that passes your lips. Be precise and honest. And email it to me for some gritty analysis if that helps you try harder.

RUTH'S FOOD DIARY: A HEALTHY DAY.

Woken at 6.30/7 a.m. by the twins after seven hours' uninter-
rupted sleep.

8 a.m.: Breakfast: two glasses of tap water; two slices of wholemeal seeded toast with butter and Vegemite, one skinny macchiato
(courtesy of my very own barista husband, Olly).

9.15 a.m.: Skinny cappuccino, shop bought.

10 a.m.: Cup of Earl Grey tea with skimmed milk.

Midday/12.30 p.m.: Lunch: two glasses of water; roast
chicken pieces (no skin) with leftover tabbouleh (see recipe on
pages 174–6) from yesterday's barbecue and half a packet of thin
green beans with a teaspoon of olive oil.

2 p.m.: Glass of water, an apple and a handful of blueberries.

3 p.m.: Cup of Earl Grey tea with skimmed milk.

5 p.m.: Twins' tea-time: snacked on soya beans (see recipe on
page 61) and one fish finger.

8 p.m.: Dinner: two glasses of water; spaghetti with meatballs,
large green salad, followed by fresh fruit salad with Greek
yoghurt.

10 p.m.: Glass of water.

11 p.m.: Bed.

A NOT-SO-HEALTHY DAY

6 a.m. start after a broken night's sleep (twin related).

7 a.m.: Breakfast: half a bagel and Vegemite; 2 glasses of water; skinny macchiato.

Drop twins at nursery, go for four-mile run in woods.

10 a.m.: Three glasses of water, skinny cappuccino and a croissant.

12.30 p.m.: Lunch with twins: Reconstructed ploughman's (cheese, ham, cherry tomatoes, raw carrot and cucumber with bagel), fresh fruit salad and Greek yoghurt.

2.30 p.m.: Another coffee (exhausted); slice of Victoria sponge cake while round at neighbours' for a play-date with the twins.

5 p.m.: Wolfed twins' leftover macaroni cheese while standing at sink, so no idea of quantity.

8 p.m.: Too tired to cook; ordered takeaway curry with a beer.

10 p.m.: Passed out.

Ruth

What I realised through participating in the diary exercise myself was not that my bad days were terrible, per se – it's just that they were more regular than I'd imagined and those healthy days were not as frequent. I was eating healthily about

50 per cent of the time, not 80 per cent. Shifting those
percentages over the course of writing this book didn't really
affect my weight, probably because I was always exercising
regularly, but it had a huge impact on Olly's. I realised this was
because most of the really bad eating was happening when we
were eating together, in the evening and at weekends.

THE GRIT DOCTOR SAYS

We have become completely saturated with dieting
information and misinformation, and the language
around food is now so faux scientific that there has
been a cultural shift away from the obvious basics
that need to be nailed before any tweaking and
finessing can take root.

It is pointless munching chia seeds all day at work if
you are eating a microwave meal when you get
home and haven't exercised all year. There is
absolutely no point whatsoever understanding the
subtleties and nuances of marathon training until
you know how to put one foot in front of the other
for half an hour every day for six months. It's the
same with food: one foot in front of the other,
reasonably healthy eating for six months or so, and

once that has become second nature, then – if you wish – you can get into the really technical stuff about things like the relative sugar content of various fruits. But don't make an impossible task for yourself from the get-go by thinking like a PhD student when you still can't read and forgetting along the way that the real crap in your diet doesn't come from bananas or pineapples or white rice but from *junk*. So back to basics, please. From the grass roots upwards, if you will – and do eat as many plants and roots as you can along the way.

Ruth

I was shocked at how much salt and saturated fat was in my diet. I was definitely one of those people who thought they didn't eat much crap. It dawned on me, guiltily, that while it wasn't strictly speaking my fault that my husband was gaining weight, it was certainly happening on my watch. I was burning it all off with my running and generally super-physical, hectic lifestyle, rewarding myself with a pie in the evening, but he wasn't doing any exercise. And what of the other stuff? I need better food to fuel all this running and twin management, not junk. My weight may be bang on but my healthy diet for life sure isn't!

EXERCISE

The Crap-Cutting Cupcake

I want you to think of what you eat as a cupcake with a cherry on the top: half of the cake represents your veggies and fruit and the other half your starchy carbs and proteins, including dairy. As long as one half is vegetable – predominantly green – how you divvy up the other half in terms of protein, starch and dairy is up to you. The cherry is your sugars, fats and oils. If you can eat like this most of the time and are exercising regularly you are going to feel fit and energised and reach a healthy weight. It may take time. But it will work.

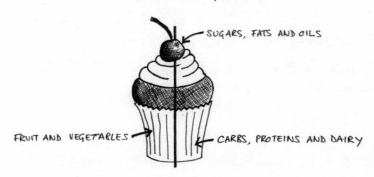

However you decide to skin this cat – and do skin it the way that suits *you* best – more fresh fruit, green veg, wholegrains, fewer fatty foods, much less refined sugar and more physical exercise is the basis for a healthy approach to managing weight – aka SAPS.

Try and commit this to memory as it contains all the information you really need.

A GRIT DOCTOR REMINDER

Covering but a minuscule proportion of the surface area of your diet – a smidgen, not a portion, nor a serving, but an artful *Masterchef* smear – are sugars, fats and oils.

The great thing about having the cupcake image in your mind is that you can readily visualise where each meal is deficient and quickly work out where your proportionalities lie and therefore where you need to make the necessary adjustments to fix things. The aim is to be *roughly right,* remember? We are not striving for perfection nor precision, just a more mindful approach to what you eat MOST OF THE TIME.[34]

THE GRIT DOCTOR SAYS

No doubt about it, sugar and fat have become the baseline of our diets. That cherry on the top is the only bit of fruit many of us are eating, and even that's sugar coated.

---

34 Remember, in Grit Doctor speak, 'most of the time' = 80 per cent of the time.

OLLY'S FOOD DIARY: PART 3

It's 23 September and Olly feels his weight is plateauing – he is still at 14 stone 3 lb. He has been saying to me that it is frustrating that he is not losing more weight and not losing it as quickly as at the beginning. Now the temptation is to try and up the ante somewhere somehow to accelerate the weight loss, but that's not my plan. Why? Because if I encourage him to go into starvation mode and try to get to his target of 13 stone 3 lb via this route, he may get there (and more quickly) but it will have been a journey through hell and he will feel as though he has crossed some imaginary finishing line. He will collapse in a 'Thank God' heap and celebrate with an industrial quantity of crisps and six pints of beer. So, this is the way I am looking at it and the way I am encouraging him to look at it: his metabolism is re-adjusting; his body is recalibrating and is now expecting better fuel: less sugar, less junk, less crap. His brain is also on board. It may take another year for the last stone to come off, and so what if it does? It took nearly twenty years for it all to pile on, after all, didn't it? If you go slowly and just make small adjustments – one Crap-Cutting Commitment at a time – you have a much better shot at remaining at that healthy weight forever. Because, once nailed, those Crap-Cutting Commitments will have morphed into good eating habits. A habit, once made, is hard to break and no longer requires conscious thought to carry out. It just happens, like getting to work on time and going for your daily run.

Olly really doesn't want all that crap any more – or at least much less frequently – because he has experienced the link between it and that photo. He is so much more mindful about eating. He often pauses before making food-related decisions. He thinks about hunger and appetite and questions himself. Bingo. Brain retrained.

PART 3

SAPS DECONSTRUCTED

5

SUGAR

SIDE EFFECTS OF TOO MUCH SUGAR IN YOUR DIET

- Chronically high insulin levels
- Heart disease
- Polycystic ovarian syndrome
- Acne
- Myopia
- Impaired immunity
- Diabetes
- Toxic liver
- Memory deficiency
- Heart failure
- Excess belly fat
- Mood swings
- Irritability

- Weight gain
- Morbid obesity

THE GRIT DOCTOR'S SUGAR MOTTO:

The less of it you eat, the less of it you miss.

Sadly, since the 1970s when the Japanese discovered how to manufacture High Fructose Corn Syrup (HFCS) cheaply from corn, it has been getting into everything. Cheap and addictive, it has been artificially engineered to be sweeter than the white stuff and consequently is a no-brainer for the food industry: shove a load of super-sweet sugar into a product and make the consumer desperate to buy more of the stuff. One only has to observe a party of toddlers after demolishing a shop-bought birthday cake to witness that sugar rush in action. And it costs next to nothing – resulting in ludicrously low-price offers that are almost impossible for the cash-strapped consumer to resist.

So, if HFCS is anywhere on a list of ingredients, put the item in question back on the shelf. You should really avoid it at all costs, and never feed it to your kids. It is – without exception – pure unadulterated filth.[35]

---

35 HFCS is variously disguised on food labels as corn sugar, corn syrup, maize syrup, glucose syrup, glucose/fructose syrup, tapioca syrup, dahlia syrup, fruit fructose, crystalline fructose, isoglucose and more.

THE GRIT DOCTOR SAYS

HFCS is a rubber stamp guarantee that the food is crap. You never see a toddler devour a whole head of broccoli and demand another with such spirited anxious need. If the label doesn't read 'sugar' or 'cane sugar', you can be pretty sure it's some form of HFCS.

The media has been advocating cutting *all* sugar from our diets and – HFCS aside – I think this is a ridiculous idea. Sugar is every bit as necessary to a good diet as anything else – it being a ready source of energy and the building block of all carbohydrates. To attempt to exclude it entirely is both unsustainable and unhealthy in my book. The natural fructose sugar found in fruits and vegetables and lactose sugar in milk and dairy products is part of a healthy diet, no question.

The real problem with our consumption of sugar is twofold:

1. The quantities of it that we are consuming
2. The type of sugars we gravitate towards, i.e. refined/processed/ HFCS/fake. Whilst there is no doubt that man-made fructose is the big bad boy of the sugar world, the white powder and fake crap we are adding to our tea and cakes is also up for culling.

THE GRIT DOCTOR WILL SEE YOU NOW

Q: But GD, how can my zero calorie sweeteners be part of the problem? Surely it is much better for me than real sugar and helping me lose weight too?

A: You could not be more wrong. Chemicals engineered in factory vats have no place in your digestive system.[36] That's the first salient point. Secondly, adding three sweeteners into your seventh mug of coffee keeps you trapped in the bad habit of wanting your coffee to taste sweet. It is a bad habit no matter how artfully it is disguised. You need to train yourself out of wanting it to taste so sweet and into savouring the flavour of non-sweetened macchiato until that non-fat milk is all the sugar hit you need.

Ruth

In the last two weeks I've had two conversations about sugar that genuinely shocked me. The first was after a memorial service as I reached for a slice of buttered fruit loaf to have with my cup of tea. My old pal from university told me I

---

36 Aspartame accounts for over 75% of the adverse reactions to food additives reported to the FDA. Many of these reactions are very serious, including seizures and death. It is widely regarded to be poisonous.

shouldn't eat it because 'sugar is bad for you' – all the while chowing down on a white bread egg-mayonnaise sandwich, clearly oblivious to the fact that he too was eating sugar. At another party, a friend commented that she ought to stop eating so many apples because they are full of sugar. This sort of conversation is utter madness and indicative of the power the diet industry and media have over us all.

EXERCISE

It ain't rocket science to distinguish between good and bad sugars. Have a look at the list below, all of which are foodstuffs containing sugar, and tick the ones you think are okay to eat and the ones you suspect are not.

THE GRIT DOCTOR SAYS
You are beyond salvation if you get any of these wrong.

- Strawberries
- Chocolate bar
- Pasta
- Haribo Tangfastics

- Bread
- Rice
- Bran flakes
- Brownies
- Apples
- Coca-cola

You see how much you know already? How your common sense screams the glaringly obvious at you?

Don't spend too much time internally debating whether pasta and bread are, in fact, good for you and how much sugar is in white rice. They are not the problem. It's the Mars bar/cream cake/apple strudel/doughnut/packet of sweets/granola bar (yes, granola bar) that's your problem.

THE GRIT DOCTOR SAYS

At this stage of the proceedings, if you are fat, take it as read that white rice is the least of your effing worries.

Confusing a crap-heavy diet with silly distinctions and distractions this early on is just another way to set yourself up to fail and is a prime example of the sort of crappy thinking that needs cutting out. When in doubt, mentally compare the snack you're tempted to devour to a packet of sweeties. Tune in to your common sense and you will have your answer. What I mean is, if you fancy a hunk of brown bread and butter and it is going to satisfy you sufficiently that you don't reach for the family-sized Galaxy bar, or whatever your poison, that counts as a massive result in my book.

THE GRIT DOCTOR SAYS

'Better than . . .' is more often than not all the crap-cutting that is required.

FRUIT IS NOT THE ENEMY

Now that the sugar conversation has extended to putting people off fruit, it has become absurd. There is never an occasion when it is bad for your health to eat fresh fruit. Nor will it ever be decreed that a banana-gobbling epidemic is responsible for making our children so fat. Get a grip. Yes, fruit contains sugar, but providing it contains (as all fruit does) so many other nutritious gems – fibre, roughage, vitamins, minerals, hydrating properties and antioxidants – it is carbohydrate fuel at its best and low in calories to boot. That fruit bowl needs to occupy pride of place in your kitchen and must be well stocked and emptied regularly. We all need sugars in our diet, and fruit is a very obvious healthy place to find them.

THE GRIT DOCTOR SAYS

It's the strawberry PAVLOVA or the orange
CHEESECAKE or the banOFFEE pie that did it, not a
denuded pear from a fruit bowl. And no one ever
got fat from eating too many root vegetables. Like
NEVER. EVER.[37]

FRUITY DISTINCTIONS

Where fresh fruit is the answer to healthy eating, fruit juice is by
contrast very much part of the problem. Production and consumption of fruit juice, fruity soft drinks and yoghurts has
rocketed alongside the advent of HFCS which is saturating them
all. Fruit was never meant to be used as a thirst-quencher and
fruit juice was historically seen as a medicinal vitamin shot.[38]
Smoothies are not much better, no matter how pretty the packaging, because when fruit is blended the insoluble fibre is lost in
the process.

---

37 <u>Once again I remind you that chips do not count as a vegetable</u>.
38 *The Care and Feeding of Children, a Catechism for the Use of Mothers and Children's Nurses*
by Holt L. Emmett. In this book from the 1920s on feeding children it was recommended
that you should give toddlers just one to four tablespoons (15–60ml) of fresh orange or
peach juice a day. Compare this with today's children's 200ml juice boxes, which contain
about 17g sugar (about four teaspoons-worth) to see how drinking habits have dramatically
changed.

People look to fruit juices as part of their five-a-day and don't take account of all the sugar. Think of it like this: common sense plainly dictates that man was not meant to consume the juice of eighteen oranges at once. This is what is so explosive about fruit drinks. *That* much sugar in one super-fast hit is going to wreak havoc on your blood-sugar levels because your liver doesn't get any time to metabolise it. And the diet varieties are just as full of crap. A cursory glance at the label of any no-added-sugar orange squash or the ingredients that make up a diet cola will be completely indecipherable such is the list of chemicals and additives and fake sugars added to make it remotely palatable.

THE GRIT DOCTOR EMPHASISES

Diet versions or sugar-free versions of foods or drinks are still not healthy. Low-fat almost always translates into high-sugar and no-added-sugar translates into chemical-ridden, man-made crap.

Probably one of the biggest changes you can make to your diet, the one that will have a massive impact on weight control and general health, is giving up all soft drinks and dramatically reducing your consumption of fruit juices – fresh, concentrated, carbonated, cordials, all of them. Even the ones with the super smart eco-friendly packaging are still crap because we are all consuming way too much of them.

THE GRIT DOCTOR SAYS

Human beings quench their thirst through drinking water. Not juice.

The World Health Organisation recommends no more than ten teaspoons of sugar a day for an adult (guidelines from 2002). More recent draft guidelines from the WHO suggest that a reduction to below 5% of total energy intake per day would have additional benefits. Five per cent of total energy intake is equivalent to around 25 grams (around 6 teaspoons) of sugar per day for an adult of normal Body Mass Index (BMI). And guess what?

- A glass of freshly squeezed orange juice can contain eight teaspoons
- A tall Starbucks caramel Frappuccino with whipped cream has eleven teaspoons
- A can of Coke has nine teaspoons
- A Pret Five Berry Bowl (fruits, yoghurt and granola) has eight and a half teaspoons
- A Mars bar has eight teaspoons

We are ladling unnecessary added sugar into our diets – the daily maximum in some cases devoured in one giant gulp before we even get to the office. Before the day has even really begun.

Ruth

It is actually really easy to wean yourself and your kids off fruit juice. Just start diluting the stuff with water and then continue to dilute it incrementally until the coloured water becomes what it was always meant to be: pure H_2O. By this stage, water should be all you and your kids will want anyway as the sweet stuff will have genuinely become unpalatable.

THE GRIT DOCTOR SAYS

With food, cook everything from scratch and when it comes to liquids, just drink water. If this is your guiding principle and you manage to follow it most of the time, you are going to dramatically reduce the crap content of your diet *effortlessly*.

SUGAR TIPS

- Work with your routine and hunger cues. Don't skip meals; this leads to a massive dip in insulin levels and feeds cravings.
- Tinned fruit is fantastically cheap, super sweet and ready to eat

in milliseconds. Always buy in its natural juices, not in syrup no matter how light. And still drain off all the juice. It is plenty sweet enough without.

- In baking recipes, use half the amount of sugar suggested. It is amazing how sweet a cake still tastes with even half the sugar. If half seems a step too far, just reduce the amount by a quarter.
- Apparently full-fat natural yoghurt makes an excellent substitute for butter in baking recipes. I've not given this a go yet, but imagine how much less calorific those cakes are going to be with half the sugar and yoghurt instead of butter.
- Fresh fruit. Nuff said about this already.
- A small slither of cake or pudding at tea-time is better than a face-full at midnight.
- The odd biscuit isn't going to kill you. A whole packet, though, just might in the long run.
- Heavy alcohol consumption is going to really ramp up your sugars and calories. Champagne is the least calorific so opt for it wherever possible! Cocktails and beer are sugar loaded. Know your poison and choose to manage it better (*note to self, Grit Doctor – err, more champagne?*).

THE GRIT DOCTOR SAYS

Compulsive buying of confectionery from the newsagents or wherever else is simply another bad habit that a bit of GRIT can break.

THE GRIT DOCTOR WILL SEE YOU NOW

Q: How can I tell if it's a bad habit that needs breaking?

A:

- You instruct family members to bulk-buy exotic foreign chocolates when on their travels . . . and remind them via email or text not to forget
- You have a 'sweetie bowl' on your coffee table outside of the festive period
- You could write a dissertation on the respective merits of different chocolate bars and sweets and know instinctively which suits what occasion/mode of transport/time of day best. Such is the depth and breadth of your knowledge you consider yourself to be something of a confection connoisseur
- If you delved into your handbag right now, there would be some chocolate or sweetie wrapper therein
- You consider yourself to have had a really healthy eating day if you haven't eaten a chocolate bar
- You engineer trips to the sweet shop (for the children) but always end up buying sweets for yourself. And stealing more off your kids . . .

If any of the above scenarios hold true for you, consider your consumption of confectionery to be a crappy element of your diet that needs cutting out.[39]

A Grit Doctor reminder: The less of this stuff you eat, the less of it you will crave.

Recipe: Sarah's banana and choc-chip loaf

When your bananas are almost over make this incredible banana and choc-chip loaf and enjoy a slice with all the family. This recipe works very well without the chocolate chips and with half the amount of sugar and no sprinkling of muscovado, just so you know! But it is sensational with them and this luxuriously decadent recipe – and its creator, Sarah Sultoon – would be most displeased to find them missing.

You will need:

175g butter
175g golden caster sugar

---

39 Consider, if it helps, that the gelatin that goes in to making most confectionery is made of boiled animal carcasses. Yum.

70g ground almonds

175g self-raising flour

2 eggs

3 very ripe bananas

100g high-quality dark or milk choc chips or half and half

Muscovado sugar

Cream the butter and sugar. Add the eggs, almonds and flour. Fold in roughly chopped bananas. Fold in choc chips. Pour into a standard loaf tin. Sprinkle muscovado sugar on top. Bake for one hour in a preheated oven at 170°C (340°F). Stick a knife in the middle and if it comes out a bit gooey still, chuck it back in for another 10–15 minutes.

Yes, a home-made cake once in a while is absolutely part of a healthy balanced lifestyle. Making it can be a fun and worthwhile activity with the kids, the kitchen smells utterly delicious and inviting and it is a treat for everyone to enjoy. It is only when cake eating is a daily staple that it becomes crap. Everything turns to crap if you either eat too much of it or buy it all ready-made. Cake made at home puts you in charge of the amount and type of sugar and fats added. Plus I find if I am involved in the preparation of it, just the smell and the act of baking makes me feel satisfied in some way so I usually want just one slice of the finished product and I am done.

It's a great idea to bake a cake when you have guests/play-dates/mums with a sweet tooth/birthdays etc. on the calendar, so the whole loaf gets demolished by lots of people in one sitting. Leftover cake is like having Satan's spawn in the kitchen and will invariably lead to a regretful late-night binge.

A GRIT DOCTOR SUGAR WARNING

Only allow yourself to start baking cakes and cookies again when you are capable of eating one slice or one cookie and then stepping away. And once you are exercising regularly. Cake and cookies a healthy **diet** do not make. But they do make up part of a healthy **lifestyle** if you enjoy them occasionally. Like pudding, they can never be a daily staple but as an occasional treat they're fine: the cherry on top of your otherwise healthy diet.

NATURAL HEALTH*IER* SWEETENERS

For natural sweet kicks try vanilla pods, cinnamon, nutmeg and allspice.[40] It's all better than the white stuff and a gazillion times

---

40 Or what about agave, honey, maple syrup, apple sauce, erythritol (the sugar alcohol found naturally in many fruits), raisins, unsweetened cocoa powder, Reb A (from the stevia plant), cranberries, dates, grapefruit for sweet *and* sour, brown rice syrup, pureed banana, milk, barley, malt extract, apricot puree, balsamic glaze . . .

better than HFCS. To curb our family's sugar intake I do a few simple things:

1. No stocking up on sugary treats for the kitchen cupboards at home: no shop bought biscuits, cakes, fruit pies or cheesecakes. If we are having people over for a meal, we cook a pudding from scratch (keeping an eye on the added sugar) or in summer we often have a whole watermelon or pineapple to finish which we just cut up and hand round. It's a great palate cleanser – simple, easy, delicious and healthy.

2. Wherever possible we go for the brown alternatives: demerara, muscovado, agave, honey. But going brown *does not mean* going wild and adding more. It's still sugar, so tiny amounts measured by the teaspoon every time, and best avoided completely wherever possible and substituted with natural non-sugar sweetening options like cinnamon, vanilla pods, nutmeg or allspice.

3. No fizzy drinks *at all*, except fizzy water as Olly loves it[41] and of course a glass or two of champagne when the occasion merits; a bottle or three when this book is finished . . .

4. No buying fruit juice or smoothies or any fruit-based squashes for the house.

5. Alcohol is of course loaded with sugar, so if that is your poison, be conscious of making a concession elsewhere; a glass of

41 Sparkling water is a great alternative if you can't stomach tap water. Just make sure it's not the flavoured stuff.

*wine instead of a chocolate mousse, for example. Limit the days
that you do drink alcohol and be mindful of how much you are
drinking on those days (note to self, Grit Doctor).*

The less of these you consume, the less of them you will crave,
remember?

I highly recommend adopting the Crap-Cutting Commitment
method with sugar. Because we have grown used to so much of
it, and because it is highly addictive, I think a cold turkey
approach sets us up for regretful binges and obsessional diet-style
thinking whereas with the CCC method we are taking on our
sugar addiction one step at a time . . .

CCC 1:   No fizzy drinks
CCC 2:   No more sugar in tea
CCC 3:   No more daily confection purchase

KICKING YOUR COKE HABIT

Coca-cola is crap culprit Numero Uno in the sugar stakes and it
really does need cutting out of our diets completely. A brief story
to illustrate my point: Recently I was all out of half-term activ-
ities on account of the pouring rain and bitter cold when I came
across this brilliant article on Facebook about Coca-Cola and saw
fit to carry out an experiment on it while gainfully employing

the twins. Apparently, cola is extremely effective at cleaning grubby tiles, so off we went to the bathroom armed with containers of the stuff. However, things soon went awry: Twin 2 and I were absorbed, on our hands and knees scrubbing away, and failed to notice that Twin 1 had left the bathroom and squirrelled himself behind the laundry basket with his Tupperware container of cola. Having guzzled the contents of the container, he was sucking the life out of the cloth he'd been using to scrub with. I'm quite sure he would have actually eaten the cloth if I hadn't found him in time. He looked extremely guilty – eyes glazed, speech slurred, begging me for more. I exaggerate – slightly – but he did scream when I told him there was no more of it to drink. He wailed 'BUT I LOVE IT, MUMMY' and wept uncontrollably for ages.

What I learned:

- Twin 1 was more deranged than usual post-cola binge. He screamed, kicked and begged for more of the black stuff and was inconsolable when denied;
- Twin 2 – usually the more deranged of the two *by miles* – was easier to manage for the rest of the day than his junked-up bro who, once his screaming fit had subsided, was difficult to please – very flat and lethargic until bedtime;
- Coca-Cola is incredibly good at cleaning the grouting on bathroom tiles. But be sure to wash it off afterwards or expect bugs and floor-licking infants . . .

Sugar is a problem for us all, not just those with weight issues. Who would have thought that those innocent-looking smoothies and organic apple juices and worthy yoghurts that we give our kids as part of their daily bread are in fact the very crap that needs cutting out? If we have sugar reduction at the heart of our healthy eating plan and remind ourselves that we all actually get more than enough sugar from fruit and vegetables before even pasta and bread – let alone fizzy drinks, milk chocolate, sweets, yoghurts, ice-creams, brownies, cookies etc. – we won't go far wrong.

THE GRIT DOCTOR SAYS

Yes, your kids need calcium, but they can get it from infinitely superior sources than sugary yoghurts. Try milk for starters. And Greek yoghurt.

OLLY'S FOOD DIARY: PART 4

1 November, 13 st 13 lb. Under 14 stone for the first time! Now the issue at hand becomes as much about never going back to being a fatso as it is about always moving forward to that healthy, settled weight range. Creating a new status quo – ever so slowly – will make it much harder to change/give up/fall off the wagon. Part of that means keeping things realistic, by which I mean if the weight is not coming off and you still feel as though you are eating very healthily, then rather than deny yourself

even more food, having to eat ever smaller portions and allowing resent-
ment to creep in so that you feel as though you are, after all, on a bloody
diet, now is the time to build in more activity. Now, this is an interesting
one for Olly because he loves his one game of five-a-side each week –
but that is it. So, what is realistic for Olly now, let me tell you, is not the
Run Fat B!tch Run routine which he dutifully embraced when I wrote the
book but gave up almost as quickly as it got published. There is
absolutely no chance I am going to be able to persuade him back into
it now that the winter is setting in. I just can't see it happening. So what
is realistic and sustainable for him, exercise-wise? For a man who
refuses to run, but who likes squash, tennis and football? We are not
members of a tennis club so that is not a realistic option at the moment,
but he does have a mate who lives nearby and is a member of a leisure
centre where they can play squash. So, using my three-times-a-week
minimum rule (read *Run Fat B!tch Run*) he needs to squeeze in two
squash games a week alongside his game of five-a-side. I put this to
him and immediately he claims it is not realistic. Fair enough, one
person's realistic is not the same as another's.

Incidentally, this is why running works so well. It takes me 35–40 minutes door to door to get out for a decent run whereas his squash or
five-a-side outings are two-hour round-trip affairs. Do the maths. Sure,
I'd far rather play tennis or squash or netball but I don't have the time to
spare at the moment and I can do five runs a week without it actually
really eating into my spare time at all. But look, no matter how evan-
gelical I am about this, I have learned since writing *RFBR* that, of course,
it isn't for everyone. And one of those exceptions would have to be my

husband, wouldn't it? So, back to Olly: I am going to try and get more exercise into the weekend too without him really realising what is happening. This is easy as pie because we have twin sons aged three, with a combined weight of seven stone.

Because Olly can see the results emerging – his belt is another notch tighter, his trousers are loosening up, his face is slimming down, the chins are diminishing – he is growing in confidence and setting a much better example to the twins, eating-wise. I feel very proud of him and he is happier with himself and more relaxed about his body. Plus with less excess weight to lug around, he is infinitely more nimble during his five-a-side games and much less tired during our weekend outings with the twins.

6

ACTIVE LIFESTYLES

A GRIT DOCTOR MOTTO

The more exercise you do, the more of it you will want to do.

A GRIT DOCTOR UTOPIA ...

A world where everybody enjoys post-run endorphin rushes, better sleep, happiness, confidence and the superior fitness that comes from regular running. The athletic clothing company Mizuno wondered what this Grit Doctor utopia might look like – a nation of runners – so they partnered with the University of North Carolina where a team of researchers found out that:

A country in which everybody runs is a country where there would be 29 million happier marriages, 5 million fewer hospital visits per year, 7 billion more hours spent outdoors, 135 million fewer hours spent watching TV per week, 63 million happier dogs and 37% more smiles.[42]

A GRIT DOCTOR FACT

The more weight you'd like to shed forever, the more of your lifestyle you will need to permanently transform. And running is one of the simplest and most powerful transformations you can embrace to that end.

Alongside the explosion in cheap fake sugars stuffed into soft drinks and yoghurts and mass-produced processed junk, there has been another equally perilous trend that serves to hugely exacerbate the impact of eating all this junk: that of sedentary living. We have become a very lazy nation indeed: schools and government (shame on you, Dave) are no longer as keen on compulsory PE, and those PE classes that do exist often lack the necessary levels of physical activity to be of any real benefit, nor are they anywhere near competitive enough. Almost entirely

42 http://greatist.com/fitness/what-if-everybody-ran

GRIT-free, in fact. Which is to miss the point of the whole exercise. Pun intended.[43]

This is a crime and given the widely recognised benefits to cognitive development of physical exercise for children, our failure to provide opportunities is actually penalising them in the classroom. We drive our kids everywhere and don't let them play out in the street, so paranoid have we become about paedophiles and murderers. And guess what? When they roll out of the car door at school each day after a faceful of Frosties, a vending machine chock-full of crap awaits them. As for the grown-ups, we are even worse. Setting a terrible example by eschewing any physical exercise, shopping online, driving everywhere and spending all our free time glued to screens. The modernisation of our home and workplace has served to deepen the problem: labour-saving gadgets and ludicrously easily available fast food – because what we *really* needed was to be able to shove junk down our gobs without even having to get up – has all contributed to unprecedented levels of inactivity.[44]

---

43 A government Public Health paper from August 2013 similarly reveals that children doing more physical activity are more likely to concentrate better in school, enjoy good relationships with classmates and display lower levels of worry, anxiety and depression. Yet over 70% of young people in the UK do not undertake the recommended level of one hour's physical activity each day; just over 20 per cent of UK children engage in more than an hour of moderate-to-vigorous physical activity per day, placing the UK 10th out of 29 OECD countries.

44 According to senior European obesity expert Hermann Toplak, as explained by Oliver Moody in his article 'British Girls Become The Fattest In Europe': *The Times*, 29 May 2014.

THE GRIT DOCTOR SAYS

With all this seemingly inescapable inactivity built into our culture, we have to be more vigilant than ever about creating movement around it.

The key to introducing exercise back into our lives is to stop looking at it as something that we need to be *into* or *interested in* or *good at* or *have the right kit for* or *be fit enough to start doing* or whatever excuse you are currently using as your reason why you just don't do it. Exercise is a *non-negotiable* component of a healthy life and so instead of focusing on all the reasons why you can't or won't do it or never have done, start thinking creatively of how you can develop this essential life skill, or risk sleepwalking your way into obesity.

THE GRIT DOCTOR WILL SEE YOU NOW

Q: But Grit Doctor, I've never exercised and I feel okay. I hate it and I always have. I am not really overweight although my kids are on the plump side.

A: If you don't exercise, your kids won't either. If you eat crap, so will they. If they see you watching telly with a microwave meal they will too. We must lead by our own example. You can't tell your kid to go outside and kick a football while you're slouched on the sofa, nor can you tell them not to drink fizzy pop while swilling it yourself. 'Feeling okay' isn't enough! I want you to be feeling A.M.A.Z.I.N.G. Which is how you are going to feel after you've read *Run Fat B!tch Run* and completed the six steps. The perfect cure for the extremely exercise averse.

Food always tastes better when combined with regular exercise, although beware of using exercise as one side of your eating equation: 'I ate a chocolate bar, therefore I must do 30 minutes on the exercise bike' is not actually terribly healthy mentally, and needless to say, 'I did 30 minutes on the exercise bike, therefore I deserve a chocolate bar' is even worse. Don't use exercise as either an excuse to eat badly or a punishment for having done so. It, like healthy eating, is a celebration of the good things in life – a strong body and a healthy heart – that fosters good appetites all round.

THE GRIT DOCTOR SAYS

Whatever healthy eating regime you adopt, the pillar supporting it all is regular exercise. The more you do of the latter the more genuine pleasure you will yield from the former and the easier you will find it to reach and remain at a healthy weight.

And before anyone says they 'don't have time to exercise', try carving out just two and a half hours from the twenty-eight hours *per week* you (if you are the 'average Brit') currently spend on the sofa glued to the television screen.[45] Same for those who claim they have no time to cook from scratch – shave off another three or four hours a week and hey presto, you still have *twenty hours of telly* left after getting regular exercise and having made every meal from scratch and sat down at a table to eat it. BAM. Job done.

To all of you exercise haters who want a life (and particularly a diet) devoid of any exercise, now is the time to re-train your brain out of this mentality.

A GRIT DOCTOR FACT

Everyone has the time to do what they choose to make a priority.

THE GRIT DOCTOR WILL SEE YOU NOW

Q: But how can I motivate myself?

A: By firmly reminding yourself of all of these gritty facts about the potential consequences of refusing to take your exercise responsibilities seriously:

45 http://www.tvlicensing.co.uk/about/media–centre/news/report-reveals-latest-uk-tv-watching-trends-NEWS35

- Coronary heart disease
- Stroke
- High blood pressure
- Breathlessness
- Flabby skin
- Low energy levels
- Stiff joints
- Osteoporosis and osteoarthritis
- Poor posture
- Weight gain
- Lower libido
- Poor role model to kids
- Leading cause of obesity in teenagers
- Infertility
- Sleep apnoea (shallow or uneven breathing during sleep)

Exercise is absolutely essential to stimulate the body's own natural maintenance and repair system and is a vital component to your overall health and wellbeing. Everything that gets worse as we get older is improved through regular exercise.

The Grit Doctor's GOLDEN RULE
Regular exercise is not an optional extra but the essential feature of a healthy lifestyle.

If you cannot abide the thought of any proper sport or really strenuous activity, then get walking. More often. For longer and with attitude. Even the exercise haters among you can do this and it will really make a difference to your overall health and attempts at successful weight management. A 60 kg person walking for thirty minutes burns up 75 calories – not bad – but a fast walk can burn 150 calories[46] so with that in mind, make walking an exercise rather than just a way to get to the shops or bus stop or from the kitchen table to the couch.

Get dressed for the job: loose clothing, good trainers or walking boots if the terrain demands, and really go for it. Leave your handbag at home and get out there for a good half-hour workout. I invite you all to turn this walking jaunt into a full-blown run by following the steps in *Run Fat B!tch Run*, but just focus on the walk for now. As in: get off your arse **right now** and go for one.

The point is that once you really get into your walking, it may make you more amenable to other more intensively aerobic options that even the mere thought of make you want to kill yourself at the moment. It is amazing how the increased fitness and stamina that regular walking brings will have you gagging for something more before long. When it does, buy *RFBR*. And if it doesn't, no matter. Stick with the walking, get committed to it. Don't get depressed about not wanting to become a

---

46 http://www.nhs.uk/Livewell/getting-started-guides/Pages/getting-started-walking.aspx

Zumba instructor or run a marathon and slump back into the sofa, defeated. March on. March up. A hill. Or two.

The most important point is if you have legs that walk you to the bus stop or your car, then you can embrace walking as a proper activity to help control your weight. So no more faffing and delaying tactics. Go for a brisk walk. And then go for another one tomorrow. (You know it's brisk enough when you feel warm and your heart rate goes up sufficiently that you can no longer lecture your dog or toddler quite so comfortably about the perils of diabetes.)

THE GRIT DOCTOR DECLARES

Walking makes your cells more receptive to insulin, which leads to better control of blood sugar: nature's own inbuilt bakery deterrent.

WALKING TIPS

- Walk home from the tube stop/train station rather than getting the bus whenever you can. Consider a heavy bag to be a bonus feature that makes you burn more calories on your way home. Indeed, do this on your way to work too and make it a habit.
- Join a walking group if this turns you on; ramble, go native . . .
- Get at least one long walk in over the weekend, a four- or five-miler – rope in your other half, kids, mates too. If the kids can't

yet walk, even better. Carrying them on a long walk will result in some serious calorie burn. I often galvanise Olly and the twins with the idea of a walk to the park, and we put the roast chicken on just before leaving. Nothing better than a Sunday roast after a good long walk. And your waistline will thank you for it. The walk that is, not the roast.

- Walk your kids to nursery or school rather than drive them, setting them up with good habits at the same time as chipping away at your own muffin top.
- Walk to the supermarket whenever possible and carry those heavy shopping bags home. This is both an aerobic and resistance workout in my book. (See also carrying heavy toddlers.)
- Sure, take the escalator – but walk *fast* up and down it.

As a general movement tip, go about your daily grind faster and with more enthusiasm, which speeds up your metabolism *and* the rate at which you are getting shit done.

TOP SUNDAY ROAST TIPS

So you've been on your long Sunday walk, and you're ready for your delicious roast. The problem with a roast dinner is not the roast dinner itself – it's all the extra crap: ladlefuls of oil, stuffing, bacon, bread sauce, plus the inevitable plate of second helpings of everything immediately afterwards, all resting in a gravy bath. Possible thirds then follow, then just one more roastie to wipe up the gravy. Then pudding. If any of this rings true for you of a Sunday, and you are overweight, listen up.

Rather than let everyone help themselves to enormous portions, plate it up like you're in a restaurant. Keep proportionality at the forefront of your mind: all those delicious greens or salad (yes, salad is an excellent idea with roast chicken) in the middle of the plate, with a roasted carrot or a roasted parsnip to one side (which makes up for the fact that I'm going to tell you to serve up just one or two roast potatoes). Or try having every other roast dinner with a grain instead of potatoes ... Go on, I dare you.

Always do fewer roast potatoes than you need because it is almost impossible to resist leftover roasties. And make them big as those tiny roasties drink more butter and oil. If it helps motivate you, bear in mind that just one small roast potato can set you back a whopping 164 calories, the calorific equivalent of a Time Out chocolate bar – *both* fingers.

Once you have dished out your portions of meat, wrap up what's left instantly and put it away so no one can have seconds and there's no nibbling during washing-up. Tell everyone what you're planning to use the leftovers for so they're not tempted to steal some – 'Oh darling, but don't you want that lovely lamb ragout/beef rendang/chicken noodle soup/fennel risotto that you love for supper tomorrow?'

And the pudding? WHAAAAT? Don't follow a roast with a pud. Totally unnecessary. Have an apple instead and if you didn't go for a long walk while the chicken was in, go for one now ...

Recipe: Chicken noodle soup

Shred leftover chicken from carcass and set aside. It doesn't matter if you only have the teensiest amount of chicken left. It's the chicken stock that is key. To that end: bring to boil chicken carcass plus wings and leave on a low simmer for 1.5–2 hours with bay leaves, peppercorns, carrot, onion and celery. Remove any scum from the surface and sieve.

Finely chop thumb-sized piece of fresh ginger and half a red chilli (minus the seeds) and add to sieved chicken stock along with 2 cloves of crushed garlic. Add a teaspoon of miso paste. Chuck in the shredded chicken if you have any and leave aside until you are 5 minutes from eating it.

At which point, bring it back to simmering point and add two bundles of dried Japanese uddon noodles or soba (available at most supermarkets – but really any other noodles will do just fine. I like these flat thin ones because they come in portion bundles already, which is handy). These noodles take 5–6 minutes to cook in the stock. So, 2 minutes in, add a bag of extra fine green beans (mangetouts and sugar snaps also both work well, or combinations of all three) and four minutes after that, serve. Add chopped fresh coriander, if you like it. DO eat immediately or the green veg will discolour and the noodles will go baggy.

For a child-friendly alternative, try a little bit of the leftover chicken cut into tiny bits, a bit of the stock to loosen everything, some tinned (drained and rinsed) sweetcorn and pasta bows – an absolute HIT for kids' tea-time.

To start shifting proportionality forever you need to transform those veggies into being *the* thing you are really looking forward to tucking into. Don't let them be a boring clump of boiled greens on the side that you have to eat to get up to your five-a-day. The pork/lamb chop/roast beef is always going to taste great but trying to focus on giving salads and veg a makeover will have you eating more of them with pleasure rather than as a chore. And then you'll find yourself quite organically reducing the size of that hunk of meat or bowl of pasta.

OTHER-THAN-WALKING EXERCISE TIPS

- I *highly* recommend running – my thrice-weekly exercise of choice.
- Mix it up, find your thang – Pilates, swimming, squash – but be realistic in choosing an exercise or sport that you are able to participate in regularly. Often when you depend on someone else (as in squash or tennis) you may find it gets missed a hell of a lot more often. My preferred exercise would undoubtedly be tennis but a) I am not a member of a club and b) it would take up a lot more time in getting to a game, playing it and getting home than a run, let alone finding someone gritty enough to enjoy playing against me . . . so, it's running for The Grit Doctor for now. *Entire family breathes enormous sigh of relief* High

intensity short twenty, ten and even seven-minute bursts of exercise are having a moment. Embrace it. Some people swear by this HIIT (High Intensity Interval Training). I got roped into a twenty-minute HIIT sesh at the gym recently and it most certainly hit the spot. The point is that something is always better than nothing on the exercise front. So get up off your arse right now and give me ten star jumps.

- Don't look for the perfect solution or an exercise that is really fun, one that you truly love. There is almost certainly no such thing. And for God's sake don't start spending loads of money on it. Start with something that is cheap – or better still, free.

THE GRIT DOCTOR SAYS

There is no point in picking synchronised swimming as your exercise if it can only ever remain a ludicrous fantasy in your head. *Get real* and find something that you can succeed in doing three times a week and then get stuck into it.

Fun, love and laughter is what you have *after* you've exercised, and *because* you have exercised, not *during* it. If you are laughing during your chosen sport, it isn't sufficiently challenging. And if it's really *really* fun, you are not taking it seriously enough.

Exercise aficionados (and I include myself in this group) are perhaps guilty of reinforcing the notion that exercise should be fun; that we leap out of bed with a smile on our face, come rain, shine, wind or snow, and relish the six-mile run ahead of us. Such thinking suggests that we are a different breed and that the exercise-averse are excluded from our gang. This is a fatal error. The crucial distinction is simply that we have accepted exercise as being essential to our wellbeing and are willing to suck it up. And trust me, we are not enjoying ourselves when we step out in the rain for an early morning jog. But we are joyous and happy and grateful in having chosen to do it and for how the rest of our day looks because we made that choice and saw it through.

Once you experience, for yourself, the numerous benefits of taking up regular exercise, you will have cultivated a lifelong habit that is hard to give up. Because it brings so much added value to the rest of your life, you will simply not be able to tolerate going back to how it was before. So get moving. Right now.

METABOLISE THIS

More activity activates your metabolism. Your metabolic rate is the speed at which your body burns up calories or fat. You don't want a sluggish metabolism, which both sedentary living and yo-yo dieting practically guarantee. Your metabolic rate changes to keep pace with weight loss, which is why it only ever makes sense to lose weight slowly. The slower the weight loss the greater the likelihood of it remaining lost.

Exercise, especially strength/resistance training, really helps speed up a slow metabolism. Don't panic at the mention of strength or resistance training as the privilege of gym members and fitness fanatics. Resistance training need not involve weights or fancy gym equipment at all. You can incorporate it into your daily activity quite effortlessly by doing any of the following:

- Push-ups, crunches and squats are ideal. Three sets of 15 reps. Or 25 reps for crunches.
- Lifting your shopping and carrying it home counts as weight training in my book. Buying online doesn't. Another reason to opt for the grittier way. Grit always adds value, remember? Always try and engage your core[47] when lifting: knees bent and keeping the back straight. It is well worth investing in a decent rucksack, by the way. Go to a running or climbing shop and get technical on their ass about it.
- When you are walking home from the train station, think of your new rucksack as weights in the gym; carry it with purpose, hold yourself up straight and engage your abdominals.

47 My Pilates teacher tells us to imagine we are trying to do up the zip of a really tight pair of jeans just out of the washing machine.

THE GRIT DOCTOR REMINDS

Running or cycling or even walking either to or from the office has to be the most obvious and simplest solution to all your fitness and exercise needs. Why don't more people do it? I have no idea but I would make it compulsory if I were CEO of any company!

METABOLISM LOWDOWN

The really key point about metabolism is that a sluggish attitude maketh a sluggish metabolism. I get very irritated by people who comment on my high energy levels, like it's a predetermined feature of my personality. Rest assured, *I am absolutely faaaarkingg knackered*. But I'm not going to let a small thing like poleaxing tiredness defeat me.

Get moving, get busy, put your back into your daily grind and you will find that your metabolism starts to speed up. Your food choices and your choices to move or not help determine your metabolic rate. So stop blaming *it* for making you fat when it is *you* making it sluggish.

SHAME YOURSELF INTO IT.

Ruth

I suffer from motivation lapses, just the same as everyone, and my number one tip for getting round such a slump is to create a situation where I basically HAVE to run. This may be as simple as putting on all my running clothes when I wake up, then taking the twins to nursery in the buggy and leaving the buggy there. I bring no handbag, phone or money with me – nothing except the front door key. This serves the run in two ways: 1) everyone can see that I am going running, so it would look extremely odd if I didn't. I am ready to run, therefore I run. 2) I have trapped myself into it. I have no other option to get home but to walk or run. And this brings me back to point one – I am ready to run, so I may as well get on with it.

This one act of 'dressing up as a runner' (or walker-with-attitude if that's where you are at) when you get out of bed is effortless. It also spares you the agony of trying to look good on the school run, transforming you from deranged-still-in-same-Breton-top-with-stale-puke-stain-mum-of-three into fit and feisty sportswoman. It provides the perfect excuse for wearing no make-up and failing to shower. And it takes all of two seconds to get dressed and be 'run-ready'.

The above translates into win, win, WIN.

Ruth

It's the same as when you get all dolled up for a party and abandon the puke-stained Breton rag for the night, looking all hot in your heels and lippy. You become that sassy pre-mum personality again. Same as getting dressed up in that smart sharp suit and putting on your wig and gown. You become the hot tri-lingual human rights barrister who will marry George Clooney. I run because I have dressed up as a runner. If I didn't turn up at nursery in my runners with nothing but the twins in the buggy and a front door key I'd almost certainly go for a coffee on the way home, maybe do some emails, and the opportunity for that run might get lost for the rest of the day because the twins need picking up at midday.

Dressing it up is not just about the clothes. It's about calling yourself on it too.

THE GRIT DOCTOR WILL SEE YOU NOW

Q: Err, what are you talking about?

A: Invent ways of making yourself accountable to take the exercise you have promised yourself you would. For example, announce in the morning to your office/workstation/secretary (lucky you)/

whoevs that you are running at lunchtime. That way
you are much less likely to duck out of it. Or, if you
are going to a friend's house for dinner in the
evening, say 'Do you mind if I have a shower at your
place because I will be running over?' Very difficult
not to when you made the grand claim and they are
already making efforts to accommodate you for
having done so.

Exercise – regular exercise – is simply another choice that we all
need to prioritise, but we can make it so much easier to achieve
success when we fit it in with our lifestyles rather than trying to
make our lifestyles fit around it.

THE GRIT DOCTOR WILL SEE YOU NOW

*Q: I am inspired! I'm going to join the gym and start
going three evenings a week after work. Is this a
good idea?*

A: No. Because you are extremely unlikely to stick
with it. It involves too many choices/obstacles/
sacrifices along the way that go outside of your
routine and lifestyle: choosing not to go straight
home after work is the first obstacle, then making

another journey to the gym, getting changed at the gym, deciding what music to listen to or what telly to watch while you work out ... not to mention the workout itself ... then getting washed and changed while you're still there and then making the journey home. This is a big chunk out of your evening which could have all been bypassed without costing you a penny. In fact, by opting to cash in your travelcard and running or cycling or walking to and from work, you would be SAVING money. People who incorporate exercise into their lives like this are so much more likely to stick with it – after all, you've got to get to work somehow.

And remember, just like the diet industry, the gym is actually banking on your failure. They are invested in it. If all its members turned up as often as they claimed they would when they first joined, there would be no space to breathe, let alone a free treadmill to use. In fact 67 per cent of people with gym memberships never show up at all, which is just how the gym likes it.[48]

---

48 http://www.statisticbrain.com/gym-membership-statistics/

THE GRIT DOCTOR SAYS

Before you complain that there is no shower at your place of work – which was the same for me in chambers – your obvious option then is running home.

Bonus features of the run/cycle home from work:

- It bypasses your desire for a snack or treat and limits your opportunities to buy one on your way home
- Creates precious 'me' time to unravel stressful thoughts from the day and problem-solve
- Totally regulates insulin at a time when we are all at risk of a sugar dip
- Will have you walking through the door fresh as a daisy and in a great mood
- A good night's sleep is practically guaranteed
- Because of all those endorphins flooding your body, if you arrive back in time to put the kids to bed, you are engulfed in waves of love so fierce you may think you have died and gone to heaven. As opposed to just wishing you had . . .
- Likewise those endorphins will neutralise any desire for petty squabbling and nit picking with your partner, so it's relationship therapy too

None of this is supposed to be easy. Those of you who read *Run Fat B!tch Run* will remember the mantra *hard is the new black*. All of this is hard. Easy is buying the processed junk food and slumping on the sofa into a saturated fat- and sugar-induced coma, hosed down with wine, pointing at the telly and laughing at someone marginally fatter than you. It takes time, patience, commitment and discipline to eat well and to establish healthy routines. None of it is easy and nor is it supposed to be fun. Trying to make all of our responsibilities fun is just another way to set ourselves up to fail. But your body and mind actually love routine and grit. They thrive on hard. On discipline. Hard is what propels us into our very best versions, so stop wasting any more of your life shirking the hard work and grit necessary to get results.

And if you don't want the results – fine – but stop whingeing about being fat and unfit and complaining that you don't like running or can't understand why you are still fat when you are eating *so* healthily and doing an aerobics class once a week. Somewhere in there is a big fat lie. Part of your cure lies in accepting the hard work necessary to bring about a lifelong shift in both your attitude and current preferred foods. Being slim, fit and exercising regularly are not quirks of fate, or determined by genetic fluke, they are in the main simply good choices made regularly. Over and over again.

ACTIVITY BUILDING TIPS

- Finding ways of building activity into your day as it is and then speeding it up is a great way to help maintain weight/get fitter without actually doing anything extra or new. So for example, for me it would mean trudging up that hill on our road with the twins in the buggy with more purpose, possibly leaving the house five minutes later to incentivise increasing my speed up the hill. Holding my body upright and concentrating on my posture, tummy tucked in, pushing from my middle and not from my shoulders, and that ten-minute buggy outing becomes a vigorous ten-minute workout (think HIIT – how very *now*).

- Similarly at the weekend, when out with Olly and the twins, chasing them on their scooters, I really put my back into it and try to think of it as a positive workout rather than resisting having to do it, feeling 'too tired' and fearing looking a bit silly. Throwing our weight into stuff with our kids makes them so happy and gets us present and in the flow so time passes much more quickly. (This is key – nearing you to the nirvana that is their bedtime and your glass of rouge.)

- When at the park, don't push the swing sluggishly with one arm whilst Twitterfering with your iPhone. Engage both those arms, conscious of maintaining your posture and chip away at those bingo wings. Pushing the twins on the swings is a serious workout for me – it actually has me out of breath and makes my arm muscles a bit sore, so I know it's working and my arms have become stronger from doing it vigorously and often.

- When at a party, especially a wedding party, dance. Not only does it mean that you have a brilliant excuse for avoiding lengthy conversations with dullards and batty uncles but you are burning off that massive feast of a meal, stimulating your happy hormones, having a laugh, flirting with your other half, toning muscles and avoiding the extra five glasses of wine you might have otherwise necked in order to listen to said dullard/batty uncle drone on. It doesn't matter if you can't dance. The worse you are at it the better, frankly, as after a certain age, there is something a tad unsavoury about an oldie that starts throwing incredible shapes. Leave that cool shit to the kids.
- If you are a stay-at-home mum or dad, your buggy is the ultimate piece of kit for resistance training. In fact every outing can count as a brilliant resistance workout if you put your back into it.

THE GRIT DOCTOR WARNS

Put your back into it – yes – but don't put your back out.

- Concentrate on your posture. If you are hunched over the buggy pushing from your arms and upper back you are doing it wrong. Push from your core.
- Push faster
- Push harder
- Push up hills

- Once you get to the playground, continue the workout. Push the swing from your core, being mindful of posture at all times and trying to keep tall and straight with the core muscles engaged. This is the area most of us mums struggle to get back into shape, so cultivating a habit of being more conscious of it is half the battle because you can strengthen and engage your abdominals whenever you go out walking, just by remembering to engage them. Try and engage your core in everything you do.
- Throw your toddler in the air and catch! Get on the trampoline in the garden and jump for ten minutes (for joy when they are finally in bed). Play aeroplanes – lie down and lift your toddler up with your feet and then do 'no hands'!, land them safely on the sofa and repeat as many times as toddler requests, improving your balance, thigh tone and core. Plus you get to lie down for a minute (almost unheard of at any other time during the day).

Ruth

The way I look at it is: I have to do this shop/go to the swings/ whatever it is that I must do with the twins that day, so I may as well get more bang for my buck and turn some of that outing into a more effective workout. I never drive to the park or anywhere else with the twins – truthfully because I am beyond shit at driving, but this is great news for my waistline. I'm fitter than ever since having the twins and it's not because I'm running more. I'm running much less than I did before I had children. But running after them keeps me in shape, which suits me much better than trying to organise an exercise session after they are in bed.

I hate the term 'stay-at-home mum', by the way – it just has a ring of lazing around about it. It's all in that word 'staying', which has got to be the least appropriate word to describe anything that happens in the day-to-day life of a mother at home with her children. There is no staying anywhere. If you can stay still for a minute that is heaven, but some days go by when I may not have actually stayed still in one spot for more than thirty seconds and have not actually sat down once. I'm not complaining, just suggesting we coin a new phrase or stop trying to bloody well define it at all. All mums are mums are mums and ultimately we all have to deal with all the responsibility that the role brings, juggle like a pro, make *sacrifices and choices daily – that we invariably never think we get right – and we should all be kinder to one another. End. Of. Rant.*

WHAT BEING ACTIVE MEANS

Active does not have to mean taking up a sport and going nuts at it three or four times a week, although it can do and it is obviously great news if it does. Just walking a lot more and building greater activity into your day, in whatever ways you can, is a great place to start.[49] I am on at least an hour of moderate activity per day (just in looking after the twins) and then probably another two hours of intensive exercise per week in the form of three runs and the odd Pilates class. Your thirty-minute fast walk counts as moderate exercise; hauling your arse from the breakfast table to the bus stop doesn't.

INACTIVITY IN ACTION

Scientists, researchers, nutritionists, doctors, governments, food manufacturers, companies with hidden pro-sugar agendas – everyone is looking for increasingly obscure reasons to explain

49 NHS guidelines recommend a minimum of 2.5 hours of moderate activity per week. I am a big fan of the NHS and defer to it on all matters medical.

the collective expansion in our waistlines – from rare genetic disorders such as Prada Willi syndrome to a 'fat' gene found in mice, to underlying metabolic issues – when the obvious culprits are staring at us in the face: thirty or forty years ago it was not uncommon to walk miles to school and to work and HFCS had not yet been invented.

We played out in the street for hours on end as children, coming home to a supper that had always been cooked from scratch because our mums didn't have any other option. We never played on screens or watched television all evening because it was quite shit most of the time and the choices were limited. And our mums were dead strict. Look, I'm not trying to hark back to the 'good old days', because those days were far from perfect, but climbing trees and sprint-dodging our mums in the garden to avoid being thrashed with a wooden spoon were excellent sources of regular exercise. Technological advances are of course a wonderful thing, but we can't ignore the very obvious links between the two: we are getting fatter because we are moving so much less, and instead of eating less because we need far fewer calories, we are eating loads more, of an infinitely crappier variety. Coffee-shop culture, soft drinks and fruit juices, smoothies and yoghurt drinks instead of an apple and a glass of water, and processed foods hiding a gazillion calories because we just want the easiest, fastest route to 'feeling' good, but we cannot be satisfied this way. Not now, not ever.

No one walks anywhere, kids are stuck indoors and everyone is glued to a screen rather than a climbing frame or rock face, and convenience foods laden with sugar and fat have exploded into our salivating gobs. And when we get thirsty from all this *vigorous* activity with the remote control or mouse, instead of going to the tap, we open a can or guzzle a carton of fruit juice without so much as twitching a muscle.

THE GRIT DOCTOR SAYS

The crap of which I speak is every bit as much about believing at a fundamental level that you can get away with sitting around on the sofa all your life never getting your heart rate up and be healthy as it is about the plastic microwave meal you scoff while watching telly.

Ruth

For me, it's the mood stabilising effect, increased resourcefulness and efficiency I seem to have at my disposal and the creativity it unlocks, that keeps me going out in the cold for a dose of 'run'. I couldn't give less of a shit about having a bikini-body, in fact I have no intention of ever being seen in a bikini again, but I do care about being alive to see my sons get married and being cheerful and energetic enough to run round after my grandchildren. Please God.

THE GRIT DOCTOR BELIEVES

The natural by-product of an increase in regular exercise is a decrease in crap consumption.

7

PROCESSED FOODS

This is an area which can be incredibly confusing because when you get really knee-deep into the subject, as I have done in writing this book, you realise that basically almost every morsel that passes your lips has been processed to a certain degree: everything in a jar or tin has been through a 'process' to get there, butter had to be churned first and loaves of bread aren't found hanging from trees, because baking is of course another process, so to attempt to eliminate *all* processed foods completely from our diets, would be wholly unrealistic.

That being said, processed foods are a *huge* part of 'problem obesity' because those supermarket staples that form part of your weekly shop – frozen pizzas, chicken nuggets, pies, lasagnes, microwave meals, bumper packs of custard creams, cakes, muffins, more treats and trifles – are created in factories, often layered up with intoxicating combinations of trans fats, sugars and salt, not to mention all the preservatives, additives, flavourings, MSG and other cheap gunk that gets added in while they make their way along the conveyor belt.

PROCESSED CRAP SIGNPOSTS

- If the list of ingredients reads more NASA experiment than foodstuff
- It doesn't even look like food
- Close your eyes and visualise its provenance. Gambolling in a field? Falling from a tree? Is that burning factory vat plastic I can smell?
- There is enough packaging to trouble your conscience and give your recycling bin a meltdown
- It can go from frozen to 'edible' in three minutes flat and calls itself shepherd's pie
- It is eye-wateringly cheap
- There are a thousand of them displayed at key points around your supermarket and they're always two for the price of one. Oh, and then there's yet another opportunity to buy them just at the tills . . .
- It pops up on your screen at the end of your online shopping order 'on offer' every time (incidentally, why are you shopping online when I told you to WALK?)

- It can double up as toilet bowl cleaner
- It makes you feel a little bit like you just had a hit of crack[50]

OLLY'S FOOD DIARY: PART 5

I made the fatal mistake recently of letting Olly go and do the supermarket shop without a list and on an empty stomach. Tip: never EVER go into a supermarket hungry and without knowing exactly what you have gone in to get.

In came the chocolate treats and unhealthy sugary snacks, a bumper packet of Flakes and four incredible cheeses. Arghhhhhh! What could I do? I didn't want to be ridiculous about it so I ate two of the Flakes – GAWD HELP ME they were good – and most of the cheese, feeling like a saint for doing him such a charitable turn. He went berserk when he looked for them so I told him that I couldn't help myself and that we probably shouldn't have those kinds of things in the house as we are all bound to gobble them up. Needless to say, he didn't drop a pound that week, but he didn't gain one either so that is good. He needs to be re-inspired and I think part of that necessitates me being nicer to him: less 'run fat bastard run', and more 'Well done, darling. You are looking so much slimmer, I'm so proud of you' as I think he needs a boost. So that is what I shall do. *Grits teeth and tries to channel the good wifey vibe*

---

50 A GD warning: No need to test drive a crack pipe just to make sure you've got this analogy nailed.

THE GRIT DOCTOR SAYS

Dramatic reduction and superior sourcing of
processed foods is an essential component of the
crap-cutting way.

The easiest way to deal with processed foods in terms of cutting
the crap out of our lives is to get into the habit of looking at a
piece of food and trying to think what processes it has been
through before it goes into your mouth, because no doubt about
it, the fewer the processes, the more readily identifiable the source –
and the closer said foodstuff is to nature, the better. Having said
that, labels are so confusing that I have given up trying to make
sense of them. The government really does need to get in the
faces of the food manufacturers and compel them to provide
clear, honest, standardised labels and listing of ingredients. For
starters though, avoid anything with red lights on the label.

Until Dave sorts this mess out, the only failsafe way to avoid
processed crap is to get into the very good habit of cooking
everything from scratch.

Ruth

*Offices are most definitely a danger zone in terms of crap
consumption, because it's guaranteed that much of the daily*

assault on your waistline is happening in your lunch break. This occurred to me today when I popped out in Westminster to grab lunch among a crowd of office workers. I looked at loads of labels and realised that many of the most popular lunchtime choices were crap disguised as healthy options. Popular fad diets will always advise against the simple sandwich for lunch, but I'm a huge fan. However, I'm afraid the only failsafe way to avoid the crap you may well end up consuming if you nip to your favourite local sandwich shop for one (of the margarine, mayo, salad cream, sweet chilli sauce variety) is to make your own.

If you must buy your lunch out, two very simple damage limitation exercises will help no end. The first is only to drink water with your lunch — no fruit juice or smoothies or any such thing. Stick to H_2O. No exceptions. The second is to have a piece of fruit instead of a packet of crisps, a brownie, a flapjack or whatever your sweet 'treat' may be. Take a closer look at the labels to get a better idea of what you are really eating and how much fat and hidden sugars are involved. Be mindful. Be suspicious. That 'healthy' granola bar may be the calorific equivalent of two chocolate bars . . .

CCC1: Only water with lunch

CCC2: Only fruit with lunch

REASONS TO GO PACKED

- It's a gazillion times cheaper
- Puts you fully in charge of the added salt, fats and sugars
- Always tastes better – no danger of a fingernail appearing in your coronation chicken (this has happened to me *shudders at memory*) or mouse droppings (remember that Mr Whippy scandal in the eighties?!)[51]
- All the money you save can go on a blow-out fabulous restaurant meal once a month (20 per cent remember is eat what you like) or on some other non-food related treat that does it for you

You are never going to be arsed to organise your packed lunch in the morning, especially if you have kids, so this requires at least a bit of thought and planning the night before, and sometimes a bit of preparation. I might add pasta to vegetable salads left over from supper and leave it all mixed up in a Tupperware container in the fridge ready to put in Olly's bag for court just before he leaves in the morning. It also makes a great picnic lunch for me and the twins. If I can be bothered, I'll make all our sandwiches the night before, using good quality frozen bread which then defrosts overnight in the fridge, so the sandwich is still super fresh (and not soggy) the next day. Whatever is in the sandwich, those vegetables must feature somewhere, either in the sandwich itself

51 Not that you would EVER be tempted to eat such processed junk . . .

or on the side, same as with your meals. Proportionality. Butter bread uber-thinly and on one slice only.

THE GRIT DOCTOR REMINDS

The key is not to overcomplicate it. The easier it is to prepare and the least mess it makes, the more likely you are to stick with it as an ongoing concern.

'FAST FOOD' IS THE ANSWER

Not the McDonald's variety, you understand (although once in a while is not going to kill you),[52] but as we are time-poor, patience-light and convenience-mad these days, we do need to adapt our eating habits to suit this cultural shift. Within reason. Fast food is actually very easy and very healthy. As a general rule of thumb, the quicker the cooking, the more nutritional value is preserved. (We do need to discount the deep fat fryer from this conversation – it may be fast, but it is not remotely healthy as well we know.) Grilling, frying in a smidgen of oil, wok stir-frying and tins of convenience food (always check sugar and salt content) can be healthy and delicious and way faster than ordering a pizza.

---

52 Once in a while means you can count the number of times you've been in the past decade, not in the last month.

Ruth

Almost anything, I've discovered (like millions more before me), can be re-hashed as a stir-fry if you rip it up, chop it up, shred it, add some chilli, garlic and ginger and swish it around in a wok on a high heat for a minute or two. Chuck in some frozen soya beans, a splash of rice wine vinegar and some fresh coriander and it's Pan Asian, man. And it's a great way to preserve any remaining goodness in leftovers and keep all the goodness in your fresh ingredients.

THE GRIT DOCTOR WILL SEE YOU NOW

Q: A Confession, Grit Doctor. I got pissed and had a kebab/McDonald's/KFC on the night bus.

A: This is not a train smash. Relax. It is incredibly boring to live like Gwyneth Paltrow.

FAST FOOD AND YOU

Use the statements below to assist in establishing whether the wrong type of fast food, aka junk food, is a problem area for you.

It matters not if:

1. You struggled to make your order, having no concept of current offers, meal deals and whether things come with fries or not
2. You couldn't remember the last time you had a junky burger, or where it was from
3. You were shocked at the saltiness of your first faceful of fries
4. You felt shifty, ashamed and/or violently sick or peculiarly hungry afterwards and wanted to go to Confession.

If this is you, there's no need to feel guilty over the odd Maccy D's lapse. Forgive yourself and move on. Maybe go for a run tomorrow to clear your head and your gut.

It does matter if:

1. Your BMI is already in the danger zone
2. Your ordering skills are so honed it's embarrassing for everyone within earshot
3. You have the exact money ready in advance
4. You are a bit peeved that your usual seat is taken
5. You know from experience that even though the last train leaves in three minutes you'll still have time to make your order, pay and catch it
6. You recognise the person serving you and he says 'Your usual?'

If any of the above scenarios apply, fast food of the wrong type is a massive problem area for you that needs cutting out. Let me help you do just that.

THE GRIT DOCTOR WILL SEE YOU NOW

Q: But how? I love a takeaway burger – it's delicious and cheap and I won't give it up!

A: You might innocently imagine that potato and oil are all that are required to make those beloved fries, but you would be sorely mistaken. Into those 'potato' fries go no fewer than seventeen ingredients including canola oil, hydrogenated soybean oil, safflower oil, natural flavour, dextrose, sodium acid pyrophosphate, citric acid, dimethylpolysiloxane (an anti-foaming agent) ... and potato. They are cooked in vegetable oil (canola oil, corn oil, soybean oil, hydrogenated soybean oil with THBQ, citric acid and dimethylpolysiloxane) and coated in salt (silicoaluminate, dextrose, potassium iodide). Many of those ingredients are hazardous to human health, including those which are genetically modified (canola oil, corn oil, soybean oil), hydrogenated (soybean oil), chemically preserved and anti-foaming (THBQ, citric acid, dimethylpolysiloxane) and artificially coloured (sodium acid pyrophosphate).[53]

53 From McDonald's Transparency Campaign of 2012

Alarm bells ringing, anyone? And I've not even started on the burger patty, which is made up of no more than 15 per cent real beef. It's not all about your girth either, dear, it's about your gut, your conscience, the planet . . .

THE GRIT DOCTOR SAYS

Think about the bigger picture *if it helps motivate you*, but continue to take the small action steps every day and remain steadfast to whichever Crap-Cutting Commitment you are currently embracing. And for today that may mean for you no McDonald's.

EXERCISE

Negative associations

Think about that name you couldn't bear to give your child, beautiful though it is, because of your associating it with someone you disliked way back when. You were able to put yourself off that name forever because of a negative association. Do the same for crappy food you want out of your life. How? Negative visualisation techniques like the one below.

EXERCISE

Fire those crisps

If you want to put yourself off crisps for life, light one over a metal tray and watch how slowly it burns and how much fat drips off it. You can get a full teaspoon of fat from just one crisp, and the smoke that comes off the blackened burning crisp is foul. Really focus on the smell, and the dripping fat and the smoke. You will feel differently about crisps forever. If you don't, email me as I have even grittier techniques up my sleeve.

FAT TAKES AGES TO BURN. Commit this gritty fact to memory.

For extra grit-factor, do the crisp burning exercise with the kids – who obviously love both fire and crisps – and put them off developing this bad habit for life. Try not to set fire to the kitchen or burn anyone in the process.

Ruth

Takeaways have always been a problem area for me. If I've been on a long run, it's the end of the week and I'm low on meal ideas and even lower on energy and motivation to do anything about it and desperate for a night off from the stove, I love nothing more than dialling in a curry or a pizza. This used to be a weekly event, almost always falling on a Friday, Saturday or Sunday evening . . . again, I realised that I wasn't putting on weight because of it but it was doing Olly's waistline no favours whatsoever. So I thought to myself, how can I turn this around without feeling like I'm giving it up? How can I make my takeaways healthier and less crapful? Is there such a thing? Portions come into it. You are always going to wolf down everything you buy, right? So buy less. Buy at least one vegetable dish. Use curry houses or takeaway joints with really high standards that boast about not using MSG. Get a thin-crust pizza with veggies rather than a deep pan with meat. And cut it down from every week to once a fortnight. These changes were both realistic and sustainable and didn't leave me feeling like I was giving up something I loved. In fact, I look forward to these treats more now they are fortnightly and relish them not as a guilty pleasure but just as a pleasure. I know that I am much more likely to succeed because the changes I have made suit me down to a T.

TIPS FOR MAKING LESS CRAPPY
BURGERS/MEATBALLS

1. Use great quality lean mince
2. Make the burgers/meatballs small. Think portion size and remember that just because it's a barbecue that shouldn't mean you eat three of everything. It's still a meal so stick to sensible portions. And remember the 'no seconds' rule.
3. Use an ice-cream scoop to make even-sized burgers.
4. Use finely chopped fresh or dried herbs like thyme and parsley.
5. Crushed garlic and finely chopped shallot or red onion add bags of flavour.
6. Use a wholemeal breadcrumb for binding.
7. Don't over combine the ingredients as this makes the meatballs very hard.
8. Barbecue or grill them to lose the extra fat that drips off.
9. If making spaghetti and meatballs, just sear them before adding to tomato passata so they can take on the tomatoey sauce and don't dry out.
10. Make your garnishes, relishes and salads plentiful and interesting and home-made.
11. If you are having a bun with the burger, it is not necessary to have potatoes as well. Have either bread *or* potatoes at the meal, not both – this is a good habit to cultivate in general.

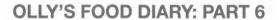

OLLY'S FOOD DIARY: PART 6

16 January 2014. Just 5 lb off target.

Very amusingly, Olly is now worried about getting 'too thin'. I'm like, 'Don't panic love, you are a long way off from that juncture!'

11 February 2014. After a bout of terrible flu and a chest infection, Olly slipped back into his old ways. It was only a bad week or ten days but he gained three pounds between the middle and end of January. Weight is staying at the same place – this has been the case for a few weeks, maybe a month now, wavering around the 13 st 7–9 lb mark and up and down and in between. Where can we make small, sustainable, impactful tweaks in his diet? Where can we improve exercise? Olly's squash partner has been away and he has not been doing any exercise other than the five-a-side once a week because even at the weekends we have often been stuck indoors in this miserable weather.

Started feeling resentful about how much cooking, shopping, cleaning etc. I have been doing for the family and being so responsible for it all *and* his weight, but decided maybe Olly needs to get more involved in the cooking and preparation? Far from this being a sacrifice for him he always really enjoyed cooking before he met me and was fond of hosting big parties – making curries and all sorts of delicious recipes learned from his mum, who is a great cook and a healthy one at that. So what happened? The Grit Doctor bulldozed her way in, insisting on being in charge of everything and then resenting everyone for crippling her with all the work. I bet if I were to say to Olly, 'Listen hon, why don't you be in charge of supper twice a week?', he'd be up for it. This way he can learn and understand about healthy eating even better, in a way that being quite literally spoon-fed is never going to teach him. I have got to take responsibility for all the complaining that I do when he would help if I just asked him nicely; he is probably keen to get into the kitchen to cook. So that's the plan. It's the morning of 11 Feb and I am going to talk to O about this when he gets home from court. Better still, I will text him: would he like to cook tonight?

BARBECUE BENEFITS

The only time-consuming part of a barbecue is getting the coals to the right temperature. Allow a good forty-five minutes or so for this. After which, anything you chuck on the barbie is fast food at its best. Barbecues turn cooking into an event, a celebration, a party – and they are entirely unavoidable if you are married to anyone with even the tiniest amount of Aussie blood in their veins. (Actually, our American neighbours also barbecue everything. I mean *everything*, and all year round.) Home made pizzas made on the barbecue for the kids to munch while the grown-ups get started on the main feast are delicious *and* nutritious in my book.

Make sure you serve plenty of gorgeous salads – like the ones I mentioned on page 61 – and pile your plate with those first before going for the meat.

Recipe: Olly's pork loin kebabs

This is a delicious, nutritious alternative to a greasy takeaway kebab, and perfect for a barbecue in the garden.

You will need:

For the raita

1 tub Greek yoghurt
½ cucumber, grated and with excess water squeezed out
1 clove garlic, finely chopped

For the kebabs

A mixture of different coloured peppers and chillies
1 tablespoon olive oil
Squeeze of lemon juice
1 pork loin
Wholemeal pitta breads

First, make the raita by simply combining all the ingredients and leaving in a bowl for the flavours to mingle.

Blacken the peppers and chillies on the barbecue, then allow to cool. Skin and de-seed the lot and slice very thinly. Put in a bowl with the olive oil and a generous squeeze of lemon. This is labour-intensive, I'm afraid, but worth it and it can be done in advance if you would rather roast them the night before.

Barbecue the loin of pork very simply, allow to rest and then slice up.

Warm the pitta breads on the barbecue while the meat is resting. Then just make up kebabs by stuffing the pittas with plenty of veg, add the sliced pork and top with a dollop of raita. Make a big one, my dear, as otherwise you will only want another and you know the 'no seconds' rule applies doubly to barbecues where everybody is a serial offender.

Recipe: Tabbouleh for 6

I often make this up for barbecues – it goes brilliantly with any grilled meat or fish and keeps well in the fridge if prepared early; just remember to leave it out to get to room temperature before eating as it doesn't taste as good very cold. It also makes excellent packed lunch material the next day for Olly. This works brilliantly with couscous – giant or small – or quinoa. And other vegetables too. I added in some blanched asparagus to our leftovers – delicious and slightly different to the day before. It does take a while to chop everything and grind the herbs and powders so well worth making a big batch . . .

I have also made infinitely more lazy versions, also delicious: leaving out any ground spices when on holiday, adapting it to suit what I've got in the fridge or herb-wise. I've used much less parsley and mint and chucked in some basil; I've also used far fewer tomatoes and instead made it with chopped cucumber. I made it recently in France with a mixture of quinoa and bulgar wheat which was delicious and I stirred through watercress and rocket leaves because I couldn't get hold of any parsley. The key really is the combination of the grains, lemon, olive oil, seasoning and fresh salad ingredients which always makes for a healthy and delicious accompaniment to meat or fish.

You will need:

60g bulgar wheat

400g ripe tomatoes

6 spring onions

2 lemons, juice only

Seasoning

¼ tsp ground allspice

¼ tsp ground cinnamon

¼ tsp ground coriander

Pinch ground nutmeg

Pinch ground cloves

Pinch ground ginger

125g flat-leaf parsley

25g mint

4 tablespoons of olive oil

Cook the bulgar wheat according to instructions on the packet. Set aside.

Meanwhile, finely chop the tomatoes and spring onions and add both to the wheat. Add the juice of 1½ lemons. Mix the spices together well, and add 1tsp to the bowl. Chop most of the stalks off the parsley, and then take a small bunch, gather together on the board and slice it as finely as you can. Repeat with the rest. Pick the leaves from the mint and do the same, being as gentle as possible.

Add the herbs to the bowl along with the oil, season and toss well. Taste and add more salt, lemon juice or spice mix to taste.

FAST FOOD: THE BOTTOM LINE

If you really must, go for a superior fast-food option and have it less frequently to make up for the increased cost. Be fast-food wise and go for the 'less crappy than . . .' choice.

Ruth

For me, as well as making those pizza and curry nights less crappy and having fewer of them, the above translates into the odd kebab from this lovely Turkish place near my house. I consider myself to have died and gone to culinary heaven when Olly brings me one home and we wash them down with an ice cold beer. Similarly, posh burger joints are cropping up all over the place at the moment: fast food, sure, but it looks and tastes like real food – no plastic in sight and the meat's provenance is declared. I know it's more expensive but I'd rather have that every couple of months than cheap, greasy takeaways once a week.

Plastic wrapping on food is an indication of the plastic, chemical-ridden fake fat and manufactured sugars loaded within. The single aim of the product? To make you want more of it and to undercut healthy alternatives.

At a really basic level, just consider for a moment what human beings ate when we were roaming around on all-fours scavenging, hunting and gathering. We went for days with nothing. It was the trees and the shrubs and the roots and the berries that formed the baseline of our diets and we really had to do an awful lot of physical work, expending vast amounts of energy, in order to capture and kill an animal or fish. I'm not going to debate here whether we are herbivores or carnivores, but what is clear is that the meat we have historically eaten came from animals that had really lived and roamed, with great muscle tone and a healthy, natural diet. They were eating grasses and plants, not factory-produced cereals designed to maximise their meat output to feed our insatiable appetite for processed junk.

SALT: THE SKINNY

For me, salt is a particular problem area that needs addressing – much as I like to kid myself that it doesn't. In 2010 cardiovascular disease caused over 50,000 premature deaths in the UK. High blood pressure is the key risk factor in cardiovascular disease and salt drives up blood pressure. The most amazing thing is that just by reducing our average salt intake by 1 gram per day, 4,147 preventable deaths would be spared each year and £288 million would be saved from NHS budgets.

And, surprise surprise, 75 per cent of the salt we consume is already added in the food we buy – just another reason why processed foods are the root of all crappy eating habits. We add another 10 per cent ourselves, from the salt cellar, and 15 per cent occurs naturally in foodstuffs. This is why, although I may add a pinch of the Maldon nectar into my Bolognese sauce, which I make from scratch, this isn't nearly as damaging as buying ready-made lasagne which already has quadruple the amount of salt in it (and that's one of the posh supermarket varieties).

Ways that I have been cutting down our salt intake:

* When shopping, getting into the habit of looking at the labelling: anything more than 1.5g per 100g is high and should be colour-coded red on the packaging. Low is 0.3g and should be green. Anything in between is obvs medium. NEVER BUY RED.

- Going easy on bacon, ham, cheddar and other hard cheeses – but don't deny yourself these exquisitely delish treats altogether. I shan't be.
- Never buying ready-made meals, which tend to be loaded with both sugar and salt. And fat.
- Cooking with less salt, using more black pepper, fresh herbs, garlic and spices to add loads of flavour with no cholesterol. Ginger, chilli, lime, lemon, curry powders, cardamom pods, pepper, dill, coriander and fennel seeds, to name but a few, pack a banging flavour punch and are kind to the waistline. Spice up your life.
- Making my own stock as often as possible as the cubes are salt heavy. Or using half a stock cube rather than a whole one.
- Making all sauces from scratch.
- Remembering almost anything in a jar is loaded with salt, so approaching with caution. Salt improves the flavour, quality and texture of food, makes it last longer and is cheap as chips (or should I say cheap as corn syrup) which is why the food industry uses it by the bucketload.
- Never buying shop-bought salad dressings, which turn healthy food into junk as soon as you open the bottle.
- Going easy on condiments like ketchup, mustard and soy sauce. Soy basically *is* salt and should be used *instead of* salt, not as well as, when making a stir-fry.

A CONDIMENT CONVERSATION

Shop-bought mayonnaise is a very bad habit. Cut it out as it's full of crap. Use full-fat Greek yoghurt as a substitute and try it out everywhere to see if it works. For example, today I made a salmon and potato salad mixing grilled salmon fillets (seasoned and covered with fennel seeds) with boiled new potatoes, artichoke hearts from an old jar lurking at the back of the fridge minus their oil, a packet of rocket, a generous squeeze of lemon and a dollop of Greek yoghurt to give it the rich, creamy consistency of an old-school potato salad. It was delicious. Half my plate was made up of that mixture and the other half was made up of broccoli.

If you always eat shop-bought mayonnaise with fish, for example, try making a salsa verde instead, or tomato concasse (see pages 181–2), and putting more effort into the flavour of your fish or potatoes or salad or whatever it is you can't bear eating without the mayo. Both these sauces go with almost any fish – the salsa verde is so punchy it does a dance in your mouth, while the tomato sauce is rich, sweet and unguent.

Look, once in a while there are certain things that must have mayonnaise, so go for home-made mayonnaise when the occasion demands. But be warned: if you are in the habit of putting the Hellmans or tommy k on the table every day, or even every other day, and you can't really eat a meal without some kind of condiment or sauce, rest assured that you are ladling unnecessary sugar, salt, fat and junk into your diet. Stop buying it until you have got this bad habit under control.

Recipe: Salsa verde

The first time I made salsa verde I used a Jamie Oliver recipe and this is basically it with a few of my own tweaks – I do it from memory as I use it so often.

You will need:

2 cloves garlic, finely chopped

1 tablespoon capers

1 tablespoon gherkins

6 anchovy fillets (optional)

2 large handfuls flat-leaf parsley

1 bunch fresh basil leaves

1 handful fresh mint leaves

1 tablespoon Dijon mustard

3 tablespoons red wine vinegar

6 tablespoons quality extra virgin olive oil

Seasoning to taste

The best way to make salsa verde is to chop everything by hand. Finely chop the garlic, capers, gherkins, anchovies and herbs and put them into a bowl. Add the mustard and vinegar, then slowly stir in the olive oil until you achieve the right consistency. If you like it with less oil – I often use less – then go for it, as that's where the calories come in.

It's great served with any fish.

Recipe: Tomato concasse

I love the word *concasse*, so that's what I call this tomatoey sauce – even though it technically isn't one. I made it on holiday recently and found myself making it over and over again every time we were eating fish. Fish can often seem dry without a butter bath, mayonnaise or some such rich accompaniment so for me this tomato concasse is the perfect compromise – much less calorific while still delivering on flavour. Rich, colourful and juicy, I put a generous dollop of this sauce in the middle of the plate and place the fish on top.

Slowly fry off chopped fresh tomatoes on a low heat (I use three large beef tomatoes but any old tomatoes will do, but use more than you think you will need as they do reduce and this sauce is delicious so you want a generous helping of it) add in finely chopped garlic (4 cloves – we were in France after all!) and a teaspoon of butter, season generously and cook slowly until the tomatoes turn orange and unguent. 20 minutes or so should do it.

EXERCISE

Processed Junk List – add your own items and think about how many may be lurking in your cupboards/freezer or on your weekly shopping list.

- Sausage rolls
- Chicken nuggets
- Pork pies
- Shop-bought pâté
- Takeaway burgers
- Supermarket ready meals
- Mayo and Tommy K
- Scotch eggs
- Ready-made quiches
- Crisps
- Cakes
- Muffins
- Cookies
- Cheap supermarket ice-cream

MAN-MADE MUCK

The combination of man–made sugars and fats along with salt makes for a lethal assault on our senses. We were not built to consume these layered engineered products and our brains do not know how to react when we do, causing us to behave like deranged addicts, unable to stop eating this rubbish or to tell when we are satiated. Processed food interferes with our brain chemistry in such a way as to make us powerless to resist the sight, the smell, even the advertising. And to crave more. And more and more. It is, of course, created with this very purpose in mind.[54] The real horror is that because it is so cheap and takes a millisecond to cook − and eat − it is going to take more than my mini-rant to persuade us all out of the habit. This is something that government and food manufacturers need to take on and if any of them want The Grit Doctor to get involved I'm in and available for gritty conversations and round-table discussions 24/7. The Food Tsar is a fictitious job title I shall now covet.

THE GRIT DOCTOR CLARIFIES

By 'man-made', just so you can get a visual on it, I am talking about chemicals combined and manipulated in huge factory vats that could not be further away from churned butter and cows.

---

54 According to *The End of Overeating* by David A. Kessler, M.D. (Rodale, 2009)

THE GRIT DOCTOR SAYS

Time spent at a chopping board and slaving over a hot stove is inevitable in your quest to cut crap out of your life. Lasagne was never meant to take three minutes to cook. It is a labour of love. That is the whole point.

The real crap are the shop-bought versions, of course. But even home-cooked varieties of rich, high-fat foods quickly become crap too if you are eating them every day. While they cease to be processed junk, they can rapidly become spectacularly calorific. Victoria Sponge should never be a daily staple even if you are milling the flour yourself. Take it as read that almost no one's sugar and fat intake is cherry-sized, so we really do need to recalibrate our bodies to consume less of them. Once you no longer depend on them in a compulsive fashion (read: having cake or a muffin or biscuit every day at tea-time) and are confident that they do represent just the cherry on your cupcake, then you will be able to enjoy them once more without guilt or fear of the damage they can do to your waistline.

Recipe: Simple tomato passata

This makes a huge batch that I freeze in portions – it's great as a base for all pasta sauces: lasagne, spag bol, sausage pasta and for pizza bases and Shepherd's pie.

You will need:

4 garlic cloves, chopped

2 celery sticks, diced

2 carrots, diced

2 onions, chopped

1 tablespoon vegetable oil

6 tins good quality plum tomatoes

1 pint water and low-sodium veg stock powder made up according
to instructions (I use Marigold) or a pint of fresh chicken stock if
you have it.

Large handful fresh basil leaves

Fry the garlic, celery, carrot and onion in the oil on a very low heat for 7 minutes or so (if you keep it on a low heat and stir often, you can get away with using even less oil). I also add a bit of leftover squash, turnip or parsnip, or anything root-related that is lurking about if it's in danger of going to waste. If I have any fresh tomatoes that need using I add those too, roughly chopped.

Then I add the quality tinned plum tomatoes (it's worth spending a few extra pennies for the best ones). Add the water and stock powder, stir, bring to a simmer and continue to gently simmer with the lid off for an hour and a half, stirring occasionally.

When the mixture is orangey and unguent, I add the fresh basil leaves and then blitz the lot with a hand-held blender so it is completely smooth.

Healthful Bolognese tips

Fry-off your leanest mince. When brown, drain all the excess fat from the pan before adding a generous splash of red wine or red wine vinegar (and allow to bubble away) then adding it all to your blended passata. (Using less mince and more tomato sauce is a surefire way to make your Bolognese more healthy.)

I season my mince with salt, pepper and a generous teaspoon or two of cinnamon powder. If you are in the habit of adding sugar or tomato ketchup (aka sugar) to Bolognese, try using finely diced carrots as in the simple recipe above, adding cinnamon to your meat and adding a mug of non-fat milk to the sauce halfway through cooking for added richness, depth and sweetness without the unnecessary calories.

Mix all the sauce you are planning to use into the pasta before serving – so not a massive wad of sauce atop the pasta, but the same one massive wad stirred into the pasta for four, mixed gently and thoroughly and then dished up. Masses of flavour without masses of sauce.

Grate parmesan on the thinnest part of your grater so that it goes further. It has a very strong flavour so there is no need to go overboard. Mindful cheese-sprinkling please.

MAKE YOUR LASAGNE HEALTHIER BY:

- Using non-fat milk in the béchamel sauce
- Using less béchamel sauce overall (i.e. not adding it to every layer) or just spreading one layer on the very top
- Using a very strong-flavoured cheese like gruyère or parmesan, or a mixture, so you can get away with using less
- Grating a pinch-worth of nutmeg for calorie-free sweetness and depth of flavour
- Adding fresh spinach or artichoke hearts to lasagne layers to ramp up the vegetable content

---

THE GRIT DOCTOR SUMMARISES

The processed variety of any food is to be shunned. But when you cook the same thing from scratch, it still needs to be aligned with your cupcake. Got it?

8

SETTLING DOWN WEIGHT

So, the idea is that after a long-standing commitment to regular exercise and a crap-cutting way of life, your body will recalibrate itself to a kind of resting place – a settling point, a weight at which it is most comfortable and likes to stay around, give or take 6 lb or so. It has always been and will always be an artificial nonsense to choose a number of pounds to lose or to pick a specific goal weight. Or be dictated to by a diet that says 'lose 7 lb in seven days' irrespective of what your starting weight is. Let your body dictate, not a book or a 'diet'. Listen to your body and drown out the nonsense coming at you from outside of it. Once you are within the normal healthy weight **range** for your gender, age and height, then settle into it and make friends with the real you.

A GRIT DOCTOR WORD OF WARNING

This weight is almost never the weight you were aiming to reach on a 'diet'. It is invariably higher.

Diets get you to chase the impossible dream: a weight which is always out of your reach. Quite deliberately too, because the industry is invested in your failure. This is the ultimate fallacy, the absolute nonsense of dieting, because it turns genuine attempts to tackle poor eating habits into vanity waistline projects destined to fail.

You cannot decide in advance what your target weight is. You can decide <u>the range</u> via an online BMI calculator. My BMI range spans nearly three stone. Somewhere within that range is where my body will choose to settle, give or take 6 lb fluctuation either way, and fighting that would be resigning myself to a lifetime of dieting.

THE GRIT DOCTOR SAYS

Give up fighting to be thinner and make friends with being yourself.

Your settling point is *your healthy* settling point, and if you are overweight or underweight, you are not currently at it and you need to re-settle yourself. Once you have been eating a normal diet and taking regular exercise for a long time (at least 6 months) then you might be approaching that point. This of course depends on how far away you were from it when you started. It is the point really at which you stop losing any weight when you are eating normally and exercising regularly.

THE GRIT DOCTOR WARNS

That you feel quite settled on the couch munching a pastry, at a stone above your recommended BMI maximum, is not the sort of 'settled' I am referring to.

The really crucial part about your 'settling down weight' is that you are built to a certain specification that – up to a point – you cannot change without going completely bonkers. This may be why that last 5 or 6 lb on any diet almost kills you to lose. Why bother, if you are within the healthy range already and clearly have wide hips and shoulders? Faaaaark it, I say. For morbidly obese crap-cutters, just getting rid of *some* of the excess weight brings massive health benefits,[55] such as reversing or preventing

---

55 'Lifestyle changes that include a healthier diet, regular physical activity, and weight loss of 7%–10% have shown phenomenal health benefits that can be more effective than medications,' says Katz, author of *What to Eat*.

diabetes, lowering blood pressure, cholesterol and triglyceride levels, improving sleep problems – not to mention having a huge impact on your self-esteem and energy levels. It is a big enough challenge just to keep *that* weight lost without adding in another vanity 6 lb into the mix. That's just unnecessary, counter-intuitive and counter-productive.

Ruth

Interestingly, Olly's weight has remained the same for the past six months, a good 6 lb or so above his 'healthy' weight range. I think this is a very positive thing and much more likely to result in his never going back to how he was before. Because just remaining at this healthier weight is hard work and it makes much more sense to get used to maintaining this weight before shrinking further into a new one that is harder to maintain and demands that he eat fewer calories. This way, his brain, his attitude and his metabolism can keep up. Slow and steady is the answer because his habits are changing (he tells me he hasn't bought a packet of sweets this year and no longer craves them at all, for example) and so is his whole lifestyle, as opposed to him embarking on some silly diet that would have him constantly 'doing battle': competing against his appetites, his instincts, while desperately clawing his way towards some artificial numerical target.

GRIT DOCTOR INDICATORS THAT YOU ARE AT YOUR HEALTHY 'SETTLED' WEIGHT

- You have to *really* try, or even starve yourself, in order to lose any more weight
- When you've had a bout of awful illness and lost several pounds, you are back to your pre-illness weight within a week without trying
- You 'feel' and 'look' exactly right. Ask your mum. Mums have a beady eye for recognising when their offspring are at the right weight
- You are operating like a well-oiled machine: sleeping soundly, exercising regularly and feeling energised. Let's call it 'optimal output'
- You feel below par when you haven't done any exercise because your body is so accustomed to getting its regular endorphin dose
- You feel satisfied by your daily bread and have stopped thinking about food in an obsessive way. You eat normally and are getting on with the rest of your life just fine
- Your weight stays roughly the same, give or take normal monthly fluctuations, and you can still wear the same dress at two consecutive Christmas office parties

THE GRIT DOCTOR WARNS

Guard against an artificially high settling point. Your settling point is never one that is overweight and reached while still eating crap and/or not exercising, excusing yourself with the 'big bones/same build as my aunt/slow metabolism/fat gene' rubbish or whatever other bullshit excuse you have been hiding behind up until now.

OLLY'S FOOD DIARY: PART 7

Olly's weight is still plateauing. Oh, and did I mention our *massive* argument when he got home last night and I thought I saw him swallowing something as he came in the door? And then he said he was full after the tiny prawn salad he'd had for lunch; too full for the delicious curried pumpkin soup I'd slaved over making – and that he knew he was having for supper. When he left half the bowl I put two and two together and knew he had snacked on something just before he came home. He exploded into a rage at being accused, then admitted it . . . and then got even more angry, claiming that he didn't have to tell me what he had eaten, that I should leave him alone. And so I bloody well did. The last thing I wanted for my supper that night was pumpkin soup, thank you very much. I'd made it with his waistline in mind, conscious that we had been away at the weekend on a culinary fest in Cornwall and had consumed a week's worth of calories. I had gone on a huge run on the Monday morning but Olly (still missing his squash partner) had done absolutely no exercise whatsoever. God only knows what he ate instead of the soup, but I was livid. I actually don't care any more about his diet and his weight; I am sick and tired of having to think about everyone else all of the time. This is never going to work unless he works this shit out for himself so that's it. I AM DONE. I have helped as much as I can and tried to set the best possible example but I have failed and I just don't have the energy to micro-manage his eating habits any more. I am not even going to ask him what he weighs. If there is anything I've learned from all this, it is that those last 5 or 6 lb can really kill one's resolve and turn 'healthy eating' into proper dieting just for the sake of losing those pounds. And it's killing me and making me despise him. God only knows how much he must hate me right now. I am not going to ask him about any of it any more or cajole him into exercise. He can be fat and unhappy for the rest of his life for all I care – ungrateful git.

PART 4

CONSOLIDATION AND CELEBRATION

9

CRAP-CUTTING KITCHEN CULL

C ongratulations. Now you know what crappy food is and just how much of it you are eating and you can visualise – using your image of that cupcake – what a healthy plate of food looks like. The time has come to treat your kitchen to a Grit Doctor-style spring clean. Applying the principle of 'the shelf', as we established in *Get Your Sh!t Together*[56], we shall do the very same with one shelf of one kitchen cupboard, but this time with less of an eye to order and cleanliness and more attention paid to the contents of each and every foodstuff. Spring clean, one shelf at a time, until your kitchen is crap free. If you are a grit aficionado and positively enjoy culls, go mental and do the whole kitchen in one go. Most cathartic. Please try not to waste food

---

56 To tackle 'the shelf' is to accept that an action must be taken in order to begin any job, and when paralysed by not knowing what that action should be, we tackle an actual kitchen shelf, and hope that our direction becomes clear during the process.

though – donate anything you no longer want and which is still in date to a local food bank.

THE GRIT DOCTOR SAYS

Relish the faecal association ('crappy' food) because it serves to reinforce a negative visual image and helps you start to turn your nose up at all this filth. When in doubt, cull.

CRAP QUALIFIERS

Getting rid of all the crap you are stocking up on in the home is a must. If it's in the fridge, freezer or any of the cupboards in the kitchen and it's crap – as defined by your Processed Junk List – it has to go. No one stands a chance if you buy crap as part of your weekly shop and stock it at home. You don't. Your other half or flatmate doesn't. And your kids do not need this crap either, no matter what lies you are telling yourself about treats and biscuits and not wanting to deprive them of sweets like you were as a child. All lies.

THE GRIT DOCTOR DECLARES

Let the crap-cutting cull begin.

Ruth

You only have to look at how we all behave around Easter time to know I'm right. Anyone with kids will know what I'm talking about. Suddenly the kitchen becomes rammed with chocolate eggs and the children so accustomed to eating them at all times of the day that it is not uncommon for them to start demanding chocolate for breakfast. And what of your own chocolate eating? Well, last Easter I was eating chocolate on a daily basis (to spare my husband and the twins, of course) just because it was there every time I opened the cupboard and the fridge. The point of all of this is not that we should ban Easter eggs and chocolate. Au contraire. Why not have a chocolate breakfast once a year? It's not going to kill you. The important point that this illuminates is how impossible it is to be healthy, and for any family members to eat healthily, unless there is only healthy food at home.

Since getting married I had resigned myself to Olly stocking up the cupboards with snacks like KitKats, custard creams, Hobnobs etc. as he made me feel that I was being a food Nazi for not allowing them. He even bought me a vintage biscuit tin which entirely seduced me into continuing to stock up on the junk to please him. But since his revelation that he wanted to lose weight, that tin has been emptied and now when the twins ask me for a treat from the tin, all they find are dried fruits or oaty flapjacks – still a huge treat in their eyes, but nothing that would tempt poor Olly. It is amazing how quickly they have stopped asking for a biscuit. I figured they will get enough of those sorts of treats when we go to other people's houses and to their grandparents, so there is absolutely no need whatsoever to keep them in the house any more.

EXERCISE

Crap qualifiers

It's your Junk List, so make it yourself. You decide, based on all that you have learned – and if in doubt email me or tweet me a pic. We are not aiming for perfection, just a healthier lifestyle and better eating habits.

A lot of crap will be lurking in the freezer so may I respectfully suggest you begin there.

THE GRIT DOCTOR SAYS

Remember, the great trade-off here is that you can eat more of what you love *if you cook it from scratch and move more in between.*

STOCK UP

As the crap-cutting way is all about nourishment and celebration, treat yourself by stocking up your fridge freezer and store cupboards with loads of good stuff. Try to buy fresh vegetables daily when you can for your evening meal. But also stock up your freezer with vegetables and fruits and save space for all those home-cooked meals you are going to be making in bulk and freezing.

In your cupboards, where before there lived ready-made sauces, tomato ketchup, sugary cereals and all sorts of sugar-addled processed junk, your cull has freed up much-needed surface area for loads of dried pasta, wholegrains, lentils and pulses. And why not broaden those horizons? There is more to grains than basmati rice. Have you tried giant couscous? When it comes to pulses, I can never be bothered to soak beans or chickpeas overnight so always buy them canned and give them a good rinse before I use them, always conscious that food in tins can be very salty and/or sugary. But adding beans, lentils and so on to stews and soups bulks them out with lean, cheap proteins and is super tasty. A great habit to get into.

Recipe: French peasant stew with leeks and beans

This is a real hit with the twins – I always make enough to save a portion for their lunch the following day. It's good for a party as it can be prepared the night before and is all the better for it.

I learned this recipe when living in France, I think from our wonderful landlady, while growing twins and writing *RFBR*!

You will need:

8 chicken thighs, skinned (and boned if you don't like the idea of
    bones floating about in the casserole, as they do here because
    some of the meat just falls off the bone)
2 tablespoons vegetable oil
6 leeks, cut into thick chunks
200g French saucisson (sometimes called 'saucisson sec' in the
    supermarket) cut into cubes
3 tablespoons of plain white flour
Handful of chopped parsley
Tablespoon of thyme
4 garlic cloves
4 bay leaves
400g can cannellini beans, drained and rinsed
1 litre hot water

Brown off the chicken in a large ovenproof saucepan or casserole dish using the vegetable oil, and set aside on kitchen towel to absorb any excess oil (if you don't have a casserole dish that can go on the hob and in the oven, just do the cooking in an ordinary saucepan and transfer everything to a lidded ovenproof dish before baking).

In the same pan, fry off the leeks and saucisson gently until softened, then add the garlic, bay leaves, thyme and flour. Stir gently and cook for a further 3–4 minutes.

Remove the leeks and set aside. Chuck the cooked chicken, beans and water into the pan.

Bake in the oven at 150°C (300°F) for an hour with the lid on.

Remove from the oven. Add the leeks back in (I remove them because I prefer them with some firmness but you can leave them in if this seems too fiddly and you like a more shredded leek!). Put the lid back on and leave on top of the hob to rest for a few minutes so that the leeks will warm through.

Sprinkle with parsley to serve. It's delicious with crusty bread and a green salad. Make sure you just have one chicken thigh each, and help yourself to plenty of the bean and leek mixture.

RECIPE REVOLVER

I heartily recommend creating a month's worth of memorised recipes for your family that you know are healthy, wholesome and nutritious and that you all love eating. Your go-to recipes, if you like. This will help enormously when it comes to ensuring your newly bare cupboards are stocked with the right healthy ingredients. You are probably doing something along these lines already quite unconsciously. But the key here is to WAKE UP, be more conscious about sugar and fat reduction and make your 'go-to' recipes healthier.

Don't make extra work for yourself. If you have a few tried-and-tested healthy recipes that you all love to eat, stick with them regularly. Too much variety is not always helpful or time-savvy, especially in the stressful early days of trying to displace bad habits. Be a stress minimiser. Variety is the spice of life but preparation and planning are the keys to losing weight, especially at the beginning. Sort your weight out first and bring the variety in later when you have a better grip on crap consumption. We have been having a stir-fry once or twice a week, a vegetarian pasta supper, a few fish nights etc. Simples. If O suggests he is bored or sick of something then I change it, but I'm not going to make unnecessary work for myself. I've got a book to write and twins to look after for goodness' sake.

PROPORTIONALITY AND PORTION SIZES

If you start getting your knickers in a twist about proportionality, an *even simpler* way of embracing the concept is just to eat slightly less of what you usually eat and try to make it a bit healthier where you can.[57] So if your breakfast routine is two slices of toast, lashings of butter and jam and a full-fat latte,

---

57 Mrs Hawkins, the young widow narrator of Muriel Spark's *A Far Cry from Kensington*, has a brilliant eating tip: 'It's easy to get thin. You eat and drink the same as always, only half. If you are handed a plate of food, leave half; if you have to help yourself, take half. After a while, if you are a perfectionist you can consume half of that again . . . I offer this advice without fee; it is included in the price of this book.'

change it to one-and-a-half slices of wholemeal toast with the tiniest amount of butter, Marmite or Vegemite instead of jam, and a skimmed-milk cappuccino. Over time these small changes will help you shift some weight and it will last forever because you won't feel the need to go back. Why? Because you are still eating exactly what you love. You have just learned about spreading butter thinly. These shifts actually stick in your brain.

You will always want to go back to your natural preferences or habits so it is much more likely that you will succeed if you try to work *with* these rather than against them. I am a toast in the morning person. So is Olly. So, rather than trying to initiate fresh fruit and yoghurt as a new thing, or muesli, or avocados or egg-white omelettes or whatever is fashionable, we stick with the old but make it better. We have really good quality wholemeal grainy bread packed with seeds, or bagels. And we are down to skimmed macchiatos and Olly is spreading his butter *so* thinly I actually hate it when he makes mine. This all helps cultivate the mindset that there is no diet because there *really is no diet*.

A GRIT DOCTOR DISTINCTION

Adopt a mindset of *give and take* to stay on target overall. This feeds into the '80 per cent healthy eating' idea. If you eat ridiculously healthy 80 per cent of the time and allow yourself treats the other 20 per cent of the time, but you find yourself dreading going back to your healthy food choices and fantasising about your 'treat day' pizza, you have turned this process into a diet and you will fail. You should be relishing what you eat *all the time* – the 80 per cent healthy stuff and the 20 per cent 'whatevs'.

So, when you've had a delicious home-cooked lasagne after a day lounging around reading the papers – utter bliss – don't follow it up the next day by eating all the leftover lasagne and redesigning your Facebook page. A healthy lifestyle does not need two consecutive days of lasagne eating and sofa surfing.

Ruth

I always make and cook two lasagnes in one go. It is time-consuming and labour intensive, so I'd rather kill a few birds with one stone. The danger with lasagne is not the portion of lasagne that you should reasonably eat, it's the three others oozing from the dish that tempt you afterwards. Seconds are a problem. Thirds – a catastrophe. I try and avoid this by getting rid of everything immediately after I've served it. I transfer leftovers into a Tupperware container and close the lid. I do the same for roast dinners and always follow them the next day with something very healthy and lean.

This is why banning seconds is so important for successful weight management. It is the one habit changer that has an enormous impact on your calorific consumption over time. For serious offenders it can *halve* it. And it is so easy to implement in that there are no complicated rules to follow, just a simple, straight-forward strategy. It may make you eat your meal more slowly and mindfully, really savouring every mouthful now you know you aren't having any more of it.

Ruth

I got into a really bad habit on this front after marrying Olly and becoming pregnant with the twins. I found myself so unbelievably hungry all the time that I made much larger portions of food so there was always seconds (for the ravenous twins within, obvs) . . . but this bad habit continued long after the twins were born when my calorific needs were much diminished. We would have loads of simple pasta suppers and I would boil the whole packet of pasta every time so we'd end up eating a huge bowl, followed by the same again as seconds, or at the very least another half portion size. This became the norm for us for ages and was partly responsible for Olly's expanding girth, because he wasn't running regularly like me. It was, of course, so easily remedied. It just involved boiling the exact amount of pasta we needed (or, dare I say it, a tiny bit less). If you're planning on saving a portion for the toddlers for their lunch the next day – which is of course an excellent idea – immediately chop it up into baby-sized pieces, put it into a Tupperware container and seal it, so that you don't have the option to chow down on the remains when you return to the kitchen to tackle the dishes.

THE GRIT DOCTOR SAYS

Yes, it counts as seconds if you are spooning it into your mouth from a casserole dish while doing the washing-up.

CURRY IT UP

Curries can be fantastic for healthy meals provided you bypass the ghee/butter/sugar/creamy coconut type ingredients and focus instead on the spices: the powerful aromatic flavours compensate for the fact that we're using less fat and sugar. Getting a curry on the go is actually one of the simplest things you can do in the kitchen. I make the basic tomato curry sauce as per the recipe below and sometimes add cooked salmon, leftover beef or lamb (whatever I've roasted on a Sunday often gets made into a curry on Monday or Tuesday) or prawns etc., etc. instead of the chicken. I add more fresh/dried/powdered chilli to make it hotter, or cinnamon, ground almonds or desiccated coconut for a milder flavour and I serve it with a mound of cucumber raita, wholemeal chapatis or brown rice.

Recipe: Basic chicken curry

You will need:

4 skinned chicken thighs, dusted in seasoned flour

1 tablespoon vegetable oil

1 onion, chopped

4 cloves garlic, sliced

2 teaspoons turmeric

2 teaspoons cumin

4 or 5 cardamom pods

Sprinkling cumin seeds

Red chilli and seeds finely chopped (or more if you like it really hot)

1 teaspoon garam masala or curry powder

Half a thumb's worth of ginger, peeled and grated or finely sliced

2 tins quality chopped tomatoes

Water

Salt and pepper

Brown off the chicken thighs in the vegetable oil in a large casserole dish. Remove from the dish and set aside.

Into that casserole dish, add the onion, cardamom seeds (from the pods), cumin seeds and chilli and cook slowly over a low heat. Add the garlic and all the spices and fry gently for a minute or two. Add the ginger, return the chicken to the dish, add the tomatoes and pour in enough water to just cover everything.

Bring to the boil and then turn down to a low simmer. Keep on a very low heat with the lid on and cook very gently for 1¾ hours. Check and stir often and add water when necessary to loosen sauce.

Serve with cucumber raita (see page 173 for recipe) and brown rice.

Once the chicken has been gobbled, there ought to be loads of curry sauce left, which makes for a fantastically delish soup the next day. I like the bits but do blitz for a smooth consistency if you prefer. Put a dollop of yoghurt on top and mop it all up with wholewheat pitta, chapattis, naan or just some crusty baguette (when in France . . .).

This curry works really well with other meats and fish. For example, you can make the basic sauce without the chicken, par-tially grill two salmon fillets (for six minutes or so) and then just break chunks of the fish into the curry sauce after its cooking time has elapsed.

10

ENJOYING MEALTIMES
WITH CHILDREN

I don't know about you, but as a harassed/haggard mother of twins, I have long since lost the art of enjoying mealtimes. But recently it got to the stage where I came to hate mealtimes so much that I had completely lost my sense of humour about it all. Something had to give or I was going to end up creating problems with the children's attitude towards food, as well my relationship with them – and I'd most probably end up divorced. A few things I learned:

1. None of it is your fault. I have twin sons who provide an excellent social experiment for nature versus nurture. They have completely different tastes, preferences and mealtime behaviours and this cannot have had anything to do with me. Turns out that bitch mum who makes you think you got it all wrong and gave up too quickly, and that's why your toddler

doesn't eat greens, just got lucky and birthed an easy eater. Her next one will be a shocker, just as yours might turn out to be fantastically greedy for all things leafy and green. Some of it – an awful lot of it – is just pot bloody luck.

2. Notwithstanding point 1, I did the following. Most invigorating:

- Burn, bin or bag any of those faaaarking irritating fussy baby and toddler cookbooks designed to make mums suicidal with feelings of failure. No one needs to refer to a cookbook for the feeding of babies or toddlers, like, evvvvveeeeer. Anything with the words julienne or fricassee or frittata . . . BURN IT. Are you kidding me? I hadn't seen or heard of an avocado until I was at least twenty-four and I certainly didn't eat prawns until adulthood. Kids don't need fancy expensive stuff and we don't need the aggro, let alone the cost of buying and preparing it before watching through our tears as it gets smeared all over the walls and floors.
- It is often said that it is important to introduce babies and toddlers to a wide range of foodstuffs to encourage healthy eating, but I say this is just another thing that makes mums depressed and is wholly unrealistic. I honestly cannot remember eating anything other than spaghetti Bolognese when I was growing up. Why on earth do kids need all this variety? Who says? We all know how obsessive and deranged toddlers can be. Unexpected or unexplained variety can bring about global meltdown in less than a millisecond in our house. I say stick to

what they like and keep feeding it to them until they are old enough to reason, unless they express an interest in trying new things. Don't set yourself and them up for another unnecessary fail in a day already rammed full of them.

- Notwithstanding the above, try to ensure that they are getting a balanced diet. By balanced I mean plenty of fresh fruit, any veg that they will eat, starch and dairy and some other protein from wherever they will take it. Not at every meal, as we ought to aim for in our own diets, but over the course of each week.[58] You know you are getting it horribly wrong if they are obese, emaciated or have rickets or some other such malnutrition-related disease. Otherwise, huge pats on the back all round for keeping them alive thus far.

- Massively simplify the cooking process. Remember that the less you cook it, the healthier it is so this is a win for you (you'll be less stressed and pissed off) and a win for the toddler (all the nutrients preserved in those raw carrots and cucumber crudités).

- Before you cook anything, think about how it would look smeared onto the floor and how long it would take to clean up. With that in mind, go for the easiest-on-you option. For example, grated cheese is a nightmare, cream cheese is easier, chunks of cheddar are even better.

- One cold meal a day was a game-changer for me. All hail the cheese ploughman's. I vary it by adding ham or chicken,

58 Penelope Leach, author of *Your Baby And Child*.

changing the cheese, the crudités, using a bagel or oatcakes etc. and I let the children feel involved in these micro-decisions. Note 'let them feel involved', which really means I am deceiving them into believing that they are in charge.

- Sandwiches – another underappreciated lifesaver. Don't feel suicidal with failure if your little darlings won't yet eat a sandwich or a reconstructed cheese ploughman's. I suffered three and a half years until mine would and have heard many mums complain of the same. Give it a try every couple of months until they gobble them up. When they do, crack open the champagne to celebrate having halved your feeding workload. You will never look back. Ham. Cheese. Cheese and Vegemite. Cheese and cucumber. Cheese and tomato. Ham and tomato. Cucumber and butter. Oooooh, so many sandwich options. Even peanut butter, when you have run out of real food or simply cannot cope at the end of a difficult day.

- When you do stumble across a combination of meat, starch and veg that they like, even love, use it and abuse it regularly, and crucially change nothing about it – not the method of preparation, nor the way it's cut and presented on whatever colour plate your OCD toddler insists on everything being served on.

- Create faux choices – as illustrated above, but worth developing. It is of course important that the little darlings get to develop their own tastes and get to have a say in what they are eating – without you becoming a slave to all their peculiar whims. This is a delicate balancing act. 'Shall we have meatballs and spaghetti or meatballs and penne?' 'Shall we have broccoli or green beans with that?' 'Shall we have brown bread and butter with our ham and cheese, or oatcakes?' 'Pear or apple?' You get my drift. With twins it is difficult to manage their very different tastes and appetites without using violence – err, I mean, faux choices.

- Make less food. The twins always seem to want more the less I put in front of them, I have no idea why. On the plus side, it means that there is no waste; no leftovers to tempt me. An oatcake and an apple or a bread roll can fill them up if they are still hungry after their macaroni cheese or whatever it was. It takes all the heat out of the experience and for that I am extremely grateful.

- Don't expect your kids to be able to go half-plate-green like the grown-ups. And don't panic if nothing green passes their lips for a week. They can get all the goodness they need from fresh fruits instead. Thank you Penelope Leach for making us all feel okay about all this. (But don't mimic their diet.)

- Begin the conversation early about what makes them strong and healthy and what is good and bad for their teeth. They love feeling like the 'know-it-all', so indulge that trait when it helps you to get them to eat well. When pudding is Greek yoghurt and fruit and they see this as a delicious treat – one that they request! – then you know you have turned an enormous corner. If ice-cream is standard pudding fare, you

217

are probably erring on the crap side of things a little. Rein it in.

- No greens, no pud: it's as simple as that. If you think this is a tad harsh, I don't give them greens they don't like nor do I give them a huge amount, but they must eat them, or at least most of them. Be reasonable, but use bribery. 'Okay, you don't have to eat everything. I'll eat that broccoli *gobbles it down with glee* and you eat this bit.' Job done.

Believe me, your kids will *love* Greek yoghurt with a teaspoon of honey and once they do, you can kiss all that sugar-riddled junk goodbye for good. Make no mistake, all yoghurt other than the full-fat Greek variety (or other full-fat natural yoghurts with no added sugar) is crap, and the kids' ones are often the most crappy of the lot. The fat-free varieties are often the worst, and are chock full of sugar. Just cutting this crap out of your kids' diet, along with fruit juice, will almost certainly get them back on the right sugar track. And failing to take this necessary step guarantees they will continue to exceed the maximum recommended daily amount, tripling it in many cases. Pre-schoolers should have no more than four teaspoons of sugar per day[59] and you'd be hard pushed to find any kids' yoghurt with fewer than four teaspoons of sugar, nor a little carton of kids' juice. That means just one yoghurt OR one fruit juice has them teetering at the maximum daily figure already. Before you've

59 According to the American Heart Association (AHA).

even left the house for nursery in the morning. You see now why they are CRAP.

THE GRIT DOCTOR WILL SEE YOU NOW

Q:Why does it matter if our kids eat all this sugar if they are still slim?

A: Because eating all that sugar can only mean that they are not getting enough calories from other more nutritious sources. Sugar does nothing for brain development or gut stimulation, and is without vitamins and roughage. It also rots their teeth and sets them up for all sorts of health problems in later life. Remember cutting the crap is not just about the fatties. A thin kid on a sugary diet is still desperately unhealthy and not getting the best start in life.

Ruth

Oh, but of course the twins don't like to eat the same stuff. One likes potatoes, the other rice; one likes ham but the other hates it. I am learning to see this as a challenge rather than as satanic intervention, and what I will not do EVER is give in to it and cook two different meals, as I'm certain that this must surely lead to another as yet unscaled level of insanity. I know one mother of four boys who pandered early on to such whims, catering relentlessly to their different palates, and she's spent a lifetime cooking four different meals each night as a result. Unsurprisingly, she ended up divorced and in therapy. Permanently. My first proper boyfriend's mum was inspiring. He was one of five sons (including twins at the end!) and she worked full time as a doctor. Mealtimes were still a huge family affair with food cooked from the garden, often piles of various food in the middle of the table to which we helped ourselves. What was left went back into the fridge and resurfaced the next day, added to something else as a new meal. So you could have more of something, less of the other, without creating more work for mum. Brilliant.

And look, the twins still love nothing more than shoving chocolate buttons down their gobs till they can't breathe, and occasionally they get them – elsewhere – but I don't use chocolate or crisps or biscuits as treats or bribes at all any more. A 'gingerbread man' made from apple, or raisins, fresh fruit and crackers are their snacks and we don't keep other stuff in the house. Then when we do go on an outing or to Grandma's, real puddings and ice-cream are always on offer, so there really is no need for me to have them too.

THE GRIT DOCTOR OWNS UP

The exception to this rule about sugar is potty training. One twin took to it without persuasion or accident. The other I am currently bribing with sugary treats so big it will be a miracle if all his teeth haven't fallen out by the time he takes his first shit . . .

EATING AS A FAMILY

I'm not remotely interested in advocating any particular 'family model'; it just happens to be where I am at and so it is the only scenario upon which I can write with any authority. As an aside, though, when I was single I loved nothing more than getting friends over for supper and cooking for them, because otherwise I stuck to a very boring eating regime which never involved sitting at a table and talking and feasting and generally tucking into the good stuff of life. So I recommend to anyone who lives on their own or lives with friends to make it a habit to do something together or get mates round at least once a week and chew the cud and enjoy whatever scrumptious food that you decide to make. It doesn't have to be expensive. Still not sold? Do it because The Grit Doctor is warning you that you will come to regret not enjoying meals with friends, and crucially, conversation, while you still had the chance.

Even though the twins are only three, we do eat together at breakfast, lunch and supper every weekend. Not only does it save me the effort of cooking a billion separate meals, it starts to encourage good manners, conversation, curiosity about food, understanding about its preparation, cleaning up afterwards, helping and all the rest. I find this approach to mealtimes a lot less stressful, plus it's a great way to foster experimentation: 'Oh no, you won't like this. It's not for children, only grown-ups like it.' And what do you know? They eat it! If for some reason they are not interested at all, fine, excuse them from the table and they invariably return ten minutes later when they hear me and Olly talking and laughing about something or other. The only downside to us all eating together is not really seasoning the food much beforehand (as a general rule of thumb it's better not to add any salt to kids' food) but Olly and I just add our own.

Ruth

Please don't get the idea that I'm there in a pinny and the twins are gobbling broccoli and everything's all happy and brilliant. Most of the time mealtimes are like the Battle of Britain and that's just getting the twins to sit down. This is extremely hard. We have a feral pair of twins, no doubt about it, but I am determined. And the more we practise it, the more it's going to stick. I've no idea if any of this is remotely helpful as I'm quite sure any sensible mum is doing this already but it was an effing revelation to me when a mum told me, 'Oh, we all eat at 6 p.m. at the weekend so that after it's done I don't have to do it all again later when the kids are in bed.'

OLLY'S FOOD DIARY: PART 8

12 April. Our relationship has definitely improved since I've got off his back and just left him to it. And I don't actually think he has gained any weight because I think he has changed on a fundamental level now. I don't think he buys packets of sweets at all any more. He makes himself a packed lunch for court, never skips breakfast, takes a couple of pieces of fruit with him and thinks before he dives in for seconds. All that awful pressure and tension (my fault entirely) has dissipated and I wouldn't be surprised if he is pretty much at 13 stone 3 lb or thereabouts when I invite him to get weighed with the GP on the 20th ... he may say no, of course. I don't want to warn him beforehand and have him crash diet just for a month so he can help the book! I want it to be genuine and I want him just to continue as he is. Interestingly, though, that first stone could not have been more easy and quick to lose. If you are really overweight, it's good news in some ways because you can lose weight very quickly by cutting out all the obvious crap. It's the more subtle crap that is harder both to identify and then to cut out. Regular exercise too, while easy for me to embrace, has been far from it for Olly.

11

THE FINAL WORD

It can never be right that you should need a pill or a powdered drink to slim down. It so obviously goes against the grain of nature that it doesn't even require argument. Nor is it realistic or sustainable to eat a perfectly balanced diet at every meal each day. Implicit in the word 'balance' is *give and take*. We will all continue to fall out of balance sometimes and we must learn not to have a shit fit when it happens. There will be some days when only a bacon buttie and a bar of sugary milk chocolate will do, and when the only thing green to pass your lips is a bottle of absinthe at 3 a.m. This is not a train smash. Enjoy those days. It is all part of a balanced life in my book. Because your balancer – that you can always rely on to bring you back to centre – is regular exercise. There is no avoiding the activity part, beeeatches. The more active you are the more you can eat and the more you will enjoy food, *and* the rest of your life. It is a no-brainer that you can no longer afford to ignore. So quit overcomplicating this and worming your way out of it and just go for a brisk walk. Right. NOW.

If your goal is a number on a set of scales, your approach to eating will always be fatally flawed. Once the emphasis moves away from a number and onto healthier food choices for life, in the long run your weight will take care of itself. We all have the power to cut the crap out of our lives, we have just forgotten how to access that power. We've been befuddled and duped and sold a lie for so long we have forgotten what the truth looks like, what it smells like, what it tastes like. And it reads like this:

GIVE UP DIETING.

TAKE UP CRAP-CUTTING COMMITMENTS

EXERCISE REGULARLY.

RUN FAT
B!TCH RUN

COOK FROM SCRATCH.

BE A SAPS QUEEN

Follow those three simple steps and your weight will settle down, no matter how fat you are or how hopeless you feel. Because all that is required is your commitment. To cutting out crap. To walking. To eating less cake. Genuine attitude shifts can only occur over the long term and develop through positive experiences. Think how many years it took for you to put this weight on. So slow down. Just keeping yourself from gaining any more weight this month would be a step in the right direction. A big step.

OLLY'S FOOD DIARY: PART 9

We have all learned along with Olly. It took him nearly a year to lose one and a half stone, so brace yourself for the long game. I know Olly will never go back to being fifteen-and-a-half stone because he just enjoys being healthier and fitter and still really loves what he eats. He now knows from a few years of experience and consistently making better choices that he operates better on a game of squash and a banana than a packet of sweets and an evening on the sofa. And I learned that my attitude to Olly and his waxing and waning motivation needed as much Grit-Doctoring as his terrible eating habits. This is a work in progress.

I had to hand this book in to my editor on 30 May 2014, so Olly got himself weighed at the GPs for accuracy on the 29th. He tells me he feels as though he has been at this weight, that he has felt the same size, for a while now and he feels at the right weight for him. To me, to be honest, he looks like he could still lose another stone but, hey ho . . . I also bet he will have lost another 6 lb before the publication date as I definitely think he could lose a bit more from his middle. But the important point is that all those health risks associated with his much higher weight are now gone. Being a few pounds, even 6 lb or even a stone overweight is nowhere near as dangerous to your body as being two or three stone over. He came back from the GPs with a slip of paper that reads . . . 13 stone 6 lbs.

Having reached this 'goal', *nothing* will change for him now. He doesn't feel the need to celebrate with sweets or cake – we went out for dinner anyway last night to celebrate finishing the book and had a feast. Olly will just carry on as before, because his new normal, his new black, is simply having cut the crap.

THE GRIT DOCTOR'S OLLY OBSERVATIONS

- There is no sign – YET – of the six pack I dreamed of
- He is scoring a lot more goals in five-a-side
- All his barrister buddies have asked him what diet he is on. To which he replies I AM NOT ON A DIET but I AM MARRIED TO THE GRIT DOCTOR SO DO THE MATH
- His clothes look great

- His cooking skills are much improved
- He hasn't bought a packet of sweets this year, so he tells me . . .
- He is trying to organise another school reunion just so he can get a photograph taken
- His energy levels have improved
- He says no to seconds – most of the time
- He sometimes says no to pudding[60]
- He feels happier and more confident
- The twins have stopped saying 'The magic word is . . . "Daddy's Fat Tummy"'
- The Grit Doctor has stopped nagging[61]
- And most important of all . . . we remain consciously coupled.

---

60 Actually that one is a lie.
61 Also a lie. I can't change my DNA.

APPENDIX: ENTERTAINING

GRIT DOCTOR DINNER PARTY TIPS

- Golden rule number one: downplay everything. Don't invite people round for a 'dinner party'. Don't call it one. It sounds very wanky and so nineties. Just invite them round for food. Or a meal. Or, more often than not round our gaff, it's for a barbie.

- Don't allow your guests to wait for more than three seconds before shoving a delicious, strongly alcoholic beverage in a sparkling clean glass into their outstretched hand (never actually *call* it a beverage obvs). No dilly-dallying. Literally: doorbell rings, 'Hi, so lovely to see you. Would you like some fizz? Gin? Wine – red or white?' Then get the correct drink to the right person without further ado. Delegate drinks prep to your 'sous' (husband/girlfriend/flatmate/other half) and help them to perfect the art. I am discovering that this can take some time –

potentially years – with husbands. But a really special first drink sets the tone for the entire evening. I recently went to supper at some vegetarian friends' pad: it was a really simple pasta affair, but the G&T I had on arrival was exquisite and I will remember that beautiful old-school glass, the mint, the quality of the Hendrick's gin singing above a splash of tonic for a long time. I can taste it now as I write.[62]

- Don't ask your guests to bring shit; it's your party so cater for it adequately. No one has time to make puddings, or skip to the supermarket to buy baguettes etc., and they will be pissed off at having been asked.

- Golden rule number two: preparation, preparation, preparation. Never ask for people's dietary requirements in advance. It panders to spoilt people's whims and gives them an opportunity to dictate the menu. 'Oh, I'm not mad about pork . . . ' or 'We're not so keen on fish . . . ' and so on. It is good for them to have their culinary horizons expanded and to try new things. This is an opportunity to educate them no less (I arrived at a supper the other night to be offered what looked like a maggot canapé. How utterly disgusting. In fact the maggoty-looking things were an obscure grain which had been scattered atop smoked salmon with lime mayo – but they really did look like maggots. Of course I ate them.) Back to the point, if there are any

---

62 Make sure your ice is clean and fresh (Yes, dirty ice has been served to a most displeased GD). A dirty glass is a quite inexcusable yet sadly frequent schoolboy error. Don't make it.

important dietary requirements your guests will let you know about them without prompting. If they don't tell you that they are vegetarian, for example, then consider the possibility that they have been gagging for some hot sausage. And don't ruin their evening by outing them.

- Don't make people sing for their supper and wait forever to be fed. All that time spent slaving over the food will be completely wasted if three hours into the evening and a bottle of wine (each) down, your guests finally sit down to your culinary masterpiece. You may as well have phoned for a pizza. Be organised. Remember golden rule number two and get your timing right.

- Make sure the lighting is kind. This is key. That means make it as dark as you can get away with while still being able to see each other and what you are doing in the kitchen. Good lighting puts everyone in the mood for love.

- There is no such thing as being overprepared. There is, however, such a thing as *looking* overprepared. Make everything look as effortless as possible. Practise looking relaxed. It is a skill. Practise it so it no longer looks practised. This requires much practice . . . basically you have to *pretend*. Don't give in to your anxious feelings and start fiddling with your hair and panting, eyes darting anxiously towards the stove, brow and palms sweating. Think SWAN. My pupil master taught me this when I was training to be a barrister and it's so true: you need to be seen to be serene and completely in control – nobody must see the frantic paddling beneath the surface. Prepare food in advance wherever possible. There is nothing worse than actually cooking rather than talking to guests. The more prep you do, and this includes table setting, cleaning, emptying the dishwasher, the better – but make it look dead casual. Everybody wants to relax and wants you to be relaxed and if your doilies have been laid out with a protractor and the candelabra are equidistant from the forks, you are not creating an atmosphere conducive to relaxation but one more akin to serial killing.

- Always put salt and pepper on the table no matter how bloody good you think your food is. People can have anxiety attacks if they are prevented from adding salt and pepper to their food.

- Have a ridiculous surfeit of booze. Or you will end up tucking into the Jagermeister and port when you run out of the good stuff . . . and paying for it with a two-day hangover.

- Mix single people with marrieds, young with old, gay with straight. Never worry about having the same number of men and women – or matching anything, for that matter. Nothing matches in our house. Not out of choice, you understand, but because so much stuff gets smashed or broken by the twins that we have a maximum of three matching items: glasses, plates . . . Mixing people up helps jolt them out of their comfort zones. Married chat is notoriously low grade and smug marrieds are the worst; I'd far rather a miserable on-the-edge-of-divorce couple any day of the week. Shake it up a bit and mix generations: before my younger sister buggered off to Australia I loved having her round for supper, always injecting a dose of youthful culture, vitality, general brilliance, enthusiasm and loveliness into the evening, forcing the rest of us dullards out of our cynical boring heads. Dancing on tables was standard at any supper she attended and seemed totally normal. Come back, sista, sista, you don't know how much I miss ya . . .

- Space out your courses – but not too much. Golden rule number two is key here. There is an optimum moment; but never rush people, never interrupt interesting chatter, never clear away while people are still eating and never seem hurried. On the flip side, get the mains out before people start licking their bowls, picking up crumbs from the floor, grabbing a Twix from their handbag or dialling for a curry.
- Don't comment on the food yourself. It will always taste slightly sub-par to you because you have spent too long around it smelling, tasting and preparing it, so don't do yourself down by pointing out its shortcomings to your guests.
- Accept compliments graciously. 'Oh, thanks' rather than 'Oh, thank God you like it. I spent a gazillion pounds and five weeks sourcing obscure ingredients online and I lost a finger when I was filleting the guinea fowl . . . '
- Always make it easy for guests to smoke and don't make them feel shit about it.

- Decide in advance where people are going to sit, having given it a lot of thought. Memorise it and when the time comes, without fuss, get them to sit there. The real art is making it look as though it is entirely unplanned and relaxed. Do not have it written down and read from it aloud, pointing at guests and instructing them where to sit. And unless it's a wedding breakfast, don't have place names written down. This is deeply unrelaxing and over-formal.
- Make sure people's wine glasses are never empty. Nothing worse than protestant drinking ethics at the supper table.
- Heating – get this right. Bodies generate warmth, as does cooking, so accommodate the potential increase in temperature. Sweating guests and a sweating chef are not God's Way.
- Allow the conversation to go anywhere and everywhere – the weirder and more controversial the chat the better. The most memorable suppers are those when the most taboo of subjects gets aired. 'Never discuss sex, politics and religion', I think etiquette decrees? Are you fucking joking? If I've gone to the bother of organising an evening of food and adult company avec grog, I want to know how the person next to me feels about the situation in Syria, cliteracy and for them to explain to me why they have a problem with the Vatican. I am not interested in house prices, catchment areas, toddler milestones and interiors (I am actually, but by day, my dears, by day). By night I want to get stuck in to the dark side.

Just in case I never get asked in whichever paper or magazine it is that asks . . .

The Grit Doctor's ideal dinner party guests would be:

Caitlin Moran: She only lives down the road so I have cunningly included her in case this book does really well and she feels honoured to be included in the list and we become local bezzies as a result. She must have unbelievably good chat if her writing is anything to go by.

Olly Weetch: Lame I know, but my husband is great company and knows a huge amount of interesting stuff which he gleans from obsessive reading of the *New Yorker*. It's cultural porn and I'm thankful for it. And him.

Mother Teresa: (Resurrected from the dead) just to see what her conversation was like. And to see how Olly deals with a real-life Catholic saint. I would sit them next to each other and secretly pray for his conversion.

Damian Lewis: Also local-ish. Because I am obsessed with his *Homeland* character and understand he is a table-tennis fiend and I would like the opportunity to whip his ass. Obviously this supper will be happening when we have moved into some sort of palace and have a table tennis table in the basement for just such evenings. A game of doubles with Olly and Mother T on the other side would be interesting. They would get thrashed of course by me and Damo, unless Mother T was able to organise some sort of divine intervention which would surely be enough to convert Olly? But I digress . . .

Michael McIntyre: Just looking at his face has me in fits. I would expect him to perform as-yet-unheard material throughout the evening that I would then judge and helpfully improve for a small fee and credit.

Why only these select few? Because the magic number for the perfect meal is six. At a round table, ideally. With six at a round table you can have everyone engaged in one conversation easily, but can equally form splinter groups of twosomes or threesomes quite effortlessly. Eight is too many and somehow makes washing up feel uber-effortful – there's never enough clean glasses and unbroken crockery, getting enough chairs requires going into the loft, and for Londoners like me eight may make your kitchen feel like a toddler soft-play area during half-term: claustrophobic.

Ruth

Just in case you are thinking 'Wow. The Grit Doctor must have amazing dinner parties.', this is sadly not the case. All my tips have been learned the hard way, from my own blunders both past and very much present. At a recent barbecue we ate so late everyone was starving and smashed and eating leftover Easter eggs from the fridge while waiting to be fed. I am deeply unrelaxing to be around, get drunk, overcook or undercook food as a matter of course, and over-fuss with a tendency to totally under-prepare yet manage to look desperately overprepared. No one gets a delicious beverage on arrival and I am always at the sink scrubbing inexplicably filthy glasses. And I nearly always end up having to ask guests to bring critical ingredients and berating myself for it. I ruined a recent meal by forcing all the guests to play a word association game which, it became quickly apparent, no one other than me was enjoying. Eventually my husband told me to shut up and all the guests then abruptly left. Reading all that I'm amazed Olly allows me to invite anyone over. Ever. You've got to admire his pluck.

I am keen to improve, though, and I have been watching and observing others who do this sort of thing really well. The 'don't ever' tips are the mistakes I routinely make. And Olly really does need to work on his getting-the-drinks-for-the-guests-quickly role.

EATING OUT

Ruth

When I go out to a restaurant, the last thing I want to do is worry about my waistline. I want to absolutely relish the experience from start to finish so I try and compensate elsewhere. Usually I will have eaten much less during the day and/or I will often go for a long run the following morning. Give and take, remember? Eating out is one of my favourite pastimes and I want to celebrate the experience from start to finish. The idea of cutting the crap out in restaurants and ordering poached chicken and steamed veg entirely misses the point of restaurant eating in my book. A chef's heart belongs to butter, and when I dine out so does mine. I want to die in a butter bath for that evening because it's a one-off, it's my cherry on top, it's life, it's awesome, and interfering with the joy of it is, frankly, sacrilegious – particularly if it's costing you a gazillion quid. Make concessions elsewhere, but not in the restaurant where the staff and your date won't thank you for it either.

This is fine if eating out is a rare treat. For those of you dining out every lunch break, you do need to be careful because – guaranteed – your calorie consumption will be far greater than you imagine. Avoid creamy sauces, say no to pudding, have fish often, and go for veggies over chips. If you are routinely calling the waiter over for more bread and olive oil/butter before you have even looked at the menu, you have a problem . . .

BIBLIOGRAPHY

On Diets and Dieting

Atkins Diet: A 14 Day Atkins Diet Plan Amanda Atkins

Slim to Win: Diet and Cookbook Rosemary Conley

The Brain Food Diet Dr Frank Ryan

The 80/10/10 Diet Dr Douglas N. Graham

Holistic Detox Dr Joshi

The No Crave Diet Dr Penny Kendall-Reed and Dr Stephen
    Reed

You Can Be Thin Marisa Peer

The GI Bikini Diet Dr Charles Clark and Maureen Clark

The Energy Glut Ian Roberts with Phil Edwards

We Want Real Food Graham Harvey

The New Raw Energy Leslie Kenton

The G.I. Handbook Barbara Ravage

Overcoming Weight Problems Jeremy Gauntlet-Gilbert and Clare
    Grace

Fight Fat after Forty Dr Pamela Peeke

Body Blitz Diet Anna Richardson

The Miracle Juice Diet Amanda Cross

The Food Doctor Ultimate Diet Ian Marber

Breaking Free From Emotional Eating Geneen Roth

*Losing It: America's Obsession with Weight and the Industry That
    Feeds It* Laura Fraser

*Rethinking Thin: The New Science of Weight Loss and the Myths
    and Realities of Dieting* Gina Kolata

*Perfect Girls, Starving Daughters: The Frightening New Normalcy
    of Hating Your Body* Courtney E. Martin

Fat Is A Feminist Issue Susie Orbach

A Far Cry From Kensington Muriel Spark

On Nutrition and Food

Calorie Counter Dr Wynnie Chan

Nutrition and Metabolism, M.J. Gibney, I. A. MacDonald
    & H. M. Roche

Food, Diet and Obesity Edited by D.J. Mela

Genetically Engineered Foods: Methods and Detection K.J. Heller

Reducing Salt in Foods D. Kincast & F. Angus

Nutrition For Dummies Carol Ann Rinzler

On Toddlers

My Baby and Child Penelope Leach

The Care and Feeding of Children, a Catechism for the Use of Mothers and Children's Nurses Holt L. Emmett

On Emotional and Mindful Eating

Eating Mindfully Susan Albers

Mindless Eating Brian Wansink

On Sugar and Processed Foods

Fat Chance: The Bitter Truth About Sugar Robert Lustig

Sugar Nation Jeff O'Connell

Appetite For Profit Michele Simon

Sugar, Salt, Fat: How The Food Giants Hooked Us Michael Moss

On Exercise

Run Fat B!tch Run Ruth Field

On Everything

Broadsheet articles, British Library Journals, trashy magazines, blogs, Facebook and the twittersphere

ACKNOWLEDGEMENTS

To my agent, Alice Saunders of LAW literary agency, and my editor Hannah Boursnell and her assistant Rhiannon Smith – you brilliant women you – thank you for giving me this marvellously gritty job. Another big thank you to everyone else at Little, Brown and Hachette Ireland for continuing to champion The Grit Doctor.

Thanks to great friends and family for culinary adventures: Anna Field and Lukas Konieczny (another day, another deygo), Adam & Nick's Achentoul pearl barley risotto, Joe and Clementine Cooke, Tords (who needs a cook?) and Mikkel Moller, Kathinka Foster, Charlotte Pilain, Alice Crawford, Tanya and Freddie Cartwright, Barnaby and Louise Oswald, Debs and Ethan Ladd, Andrew Bredon (spelt it right this time dude – for maggot canapes and the rest), Alice Haddon and Jean-Paul Van Cauwelaert (for sensational dukka and *that* G&T), Cameron Hill and Jason Davidson, Cara – for fine dining – and Ruaridh Brown-Hovelt, Roger and Louise Lamberth (for the chickpea recipe and wonderful summer barbeque), Sarah Sultoon, Clare and Chris Drury-Axford (for Michelin starred dps), Zoe and Andy Gordon; Zoe's parents, Jill and David Montagu-Smith for providing me with a writing haven, To everyone at Feast Deli in Muswell Hill: I still love coming to work. To Alicja and Iza for all your help in keeping the twins – and the mess – under control.

To my bigger, but better, half – Olly – thank you for being so enthusiastic about everything I cook and for being such a Saint. And my darling mum, thank you for making the best cakes and puddings in the world – from scratch.